CW00433502

SLOW LIFE DIET
GREEK VILLAGE LIVING

The Pathway to a Healthier Lifestyle, Healthy Habits, and a Happier You

STRATIS KAMATSOS

ACKNOWLEDGMENTS

I would like to express my sincere thanks to Gyorgyi and Cindy who assisted with the editing and proofreading. To Tomas and Yianni for the design and illustration of the book cover. And to Stratis M. for allowing me to use his wonderful photos. Thank you.

DEDICATION

To Gyorgyi, Stelli, and George

ONE FOR ONE PROMISE

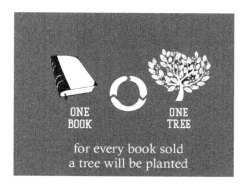

I have partnered up with Eden Reforestation Projects, as I have with my olive oil business, to continue my quest to plant as many trees as possible.

Therefore, I pledge that for every book sold, a tree will be planted in a deforested area in Africa or Haiti while creating employment for people in these impoverished areas. For every 10 trees are planted, one work day is created. The more that this book spreads and gets read, then the more we can help people and the planet.

Copyright © 2022 by Stratis Kamatsos
All rights reserved, except for those granted under copyright law
and "fair-use" provisions.

Cover art © 2022 by Tomas Watson
All rights reserved.

Illustration © 2022 by Kreativek
All rights reserved.

Cover photos 1, 3, and 4 from top left to right and inner book
© 2022 by Stratis Makrodoulis
All rights reserved. Used with permission.
All shot on location on Lesvos

4

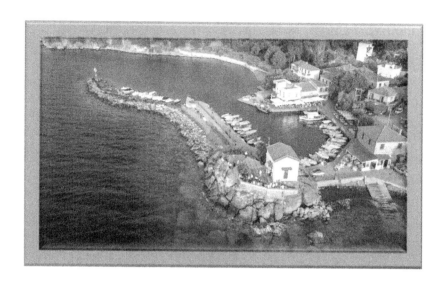

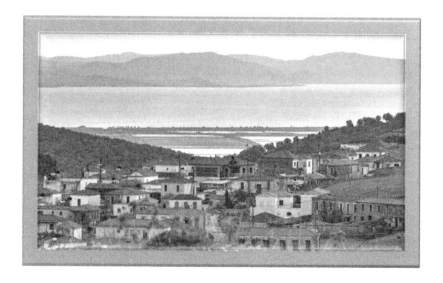

e passes, the sun settles into that perfect position. single beam of light peaks through the shutters and s upon sleepy eyes, gently nudging them awake.

Before you even enter the kitchen, the aromas wafting through the house, devilishly entice the senses. It is a house built in 1893, showing signs of harmonious wear on its sturdy foundation, like wrinkles on an elderly face.

On the table, a bouquet with an array of food, all locally sourced, rich in taste, and bursting with colors and flavor. The whole family is about to partake in an unchoreographed, allegro symphony.

After breakfast, a stroll into the center of the village, through the small alleyways that flow, like hidden tributaries, to the main river. The livestock you meet along the way greet you in a frantic but friendly way.

The main street is glittered with all the necessities one needs in a village, and the first stop is at the fishmonger to see the daily catch. Then the bakery and the local grocery shop. Along the way, meetings with familiar faces that relate the daily news like a well-oiled assembly line.

After a fulfilling *meze* style lunch[1], a collective, unofficial time for rest is declared and a hush blankets the village. The church bell chimes twice to indicate the time and to

---

[1] Meze is a selection of small dishes usually served as appetizers but could be a main meal when sharing many of these dishes.

give warning like a disciplined teacher. The weary heads rest upon feathery pillows that smell of jasmine and the fresh summer breeze; they fall into a slumber as the wind gently rustles the leaves of the olive trees and the in-tune cicadas buzz away.

The gentle, afternoon breeze prods the battered shutters, which start to creak on their rusted hinges, setting off a unique alarm. Rested eyes awaken and bodies famished craving an afternoon delight. Succulent, vibrant, seasonal fruit are laid out on the table ready to be devoured.

The sun punches out after a long day's work as the moon takes on the duty of illuminating the night, allowing the villagers to gather at the alley corners, amongst the primrose scented night air, recounting the days' events with discussions and laughter.

"Like the village...nowhere else," a common Greek saying goes. There is a reason why Greeks hold their village close to their hearts, regardless of whether they are living in a city or in another country. All of life's lessons can be learned and implemented from things found in the Greek village.

They say a picture is worth a thousand words, but an experience makes those words eternal. These memories, these experiences, were my memories, my experiences. Although having been born and raised in the United States, my parents, without fail, made a vow to themselves, and to the Greek motherland, that my siblings and I would not only be acquainted with our

Greek heritage, but also to live and experience it as a primary source. Every summer for twelve years, for an entire three months, I would be immersed in rich, village culture, going back to the roots, steeped in history and tradition. And this immersion, and the building of these foundational habits, did not stop when we departed Lesvos; these were also incorporated in our lives even back in the States becoming even more intertwined in our upbringing.

The experiences of daily life set the tone to establishing healthy habits and a healthy lifestyle that evolve from slow living. And, although it would be beneficial for one to experience living in a Greek village for an extended period of time, it is by no means a prerequisite for you to fully embrace and implement these healthy habits in your own life.

Greeks have learned these habits because they are incorporated in their way of life. They are intertwined and inherently taught to next generations who also learn from and perfect them. What is great about these habits is that it is not difficult to implement them in one's life; you will see many of them are already a part of your life in one form or another. Tweaking them or adding to them is not only possible but also welcomed. By making them your own, it may help in the adaptation transition period. Therefore, do not get disheartened with feelings of despair and impossibility before we even embark on our journey.

The hardest thing about making a true change to your life, a meaningful change that will lead to getting healthy, is actually getting started. And remember, everything is impossible until you do it.

Healthy Living

Youth is a Gift of Nature, but Age is a Work of Art[2]

When we are put in this world, we are given a gift: the gift of life. When we are young, we do not realize how precious this gift is, and as a consequence, we live with the perception that old age is a distant and far off idea, something we do not need to care about now. We also do not think about wasting time because we consider time an infinite resource that we are entitled to. However, we reach the latter part of our life faster than we comprehend, and sometimes with little or nothing to show for it, and we find ourselves desperate to extend our years (or turn back the clock) so we can still experience the things we hold so dear and we once took for granted.

Each of us are different in the way we handle and respond to reaching this part of our life. But, reaching these crossroads is inevitable, and therefore, the only thing you can do is accept this premise: we will get old. The idea is to make a plan for the best way to age.

----

[2] Stanislaw Jerzy Lec quote

Getting old simply means that your body is slowly giving way to the wear and tear of long usage, but our brain, mentally, can stay young forever. The Greek villagers never forget this notion that progressing through ages is a physical metamorphosis rather than a mental one.

Throughout the world, especially in Greece and the rest of the Mediterranean countries, families teach their children to value and respect their elders, and more specifically, the knowledge and wisdom that these elders have attained over the many years they have experienced. This idea is portrayed rather magnificently by this quote: "If elders could bequeath their experience and knowledge of life to children without the children making any mistakes, they would save them from a lifetime of heartaches".[3] If you sit and listen to these elders, one of the common themes you learn from them is that there are two things they place above everything else – their health and the happiness of a fulfilled life. These are the two things that mean the most to them at the end of their lives, and health is something finite.

With this book, I would like not only to share my experience, but also to pass on the knowledge I have obtained from living in a Greek village and observing and talking to the older generation with these two specific themes in mind: health and happiness. It is the simplicity of the way people live in a Greek village that creates such a powerful and effective way to lead one's

---

[3] Neena Brar

life in a healthier way and reach a place of contentment and peace.

An important part of this healthy lifestyle is that in Greece, the villagers have a sense of purpose, and as said above, this purpose is instilled from a young age. Their purpose is not filled with images of hobbies or playing golf when retiring, but it usually has something that not only helps themselves, but also their families, and in a broader sense, the community. It is this sense of responsibility and social utility that drives their purpose forward until they get old.

We all have our personal crusade which we face every day, trying to conquer it or faltering and giving in. For some of you, this crusade could be something small yet personal: losing weight to again fit into that piece of clothing that has been sitting in your closet for years, staring and judging you every single day; it could be about being stuck in the rat race, not living a healthy life, and waking up just to drudge through a day of routine and not having any time for yourself; it could relate to stress about your personal life, finances, or appearance; or it could just be about not having a sense of purpose or set goals in your life. There are a lot of intimidating barriers that prevent you from taking the first steps. When you finally do take them, you may feel an inexplicable (or at least it feels like it is inexplicable) resistance in not only pushing through the initial phase, but also to sticking with your new healthier lifestyle and/or exercise.

No matter what this personal strife is, no matter how monotonous and routine your life may feel, the path to surmounting this is difficult for everyone. This book aims to help you remove these intimidating barriers to entry and offer a fun, exciting, and proven way to change your life: the Greek village way of life. The secrets found in the village are presented in few simple steps, and by the end of your achieving period, you will see amazing results.

Who is this book for?

The simple answer is for the people who want to change lifestyles because the Greek village way of life is more than just what to eat. It is a lifestyle, which encompasses every aspect of the way you live your life. Thus, lifestyle is not just a fad diet. It is about understanding habits and psychology and how they relate to you, your current mindset, and the result it has on your weight issues. If you are someone who is not ready to make a crucial change to their lifestyle, to embrace ideas that will create long-term positive changes to the way you live, and to keep implementing them beyond your initial phase of excitement of trying something new, then it is best that you do not read further than this point. The 'fast fad' and the 'I want the results now' mentality is a hinderance to you making this change to the way you live.

I'm sure that most of you, if not all of you, who are still reading, have tried and/or implemented some kind of 'get results fast' diet. Some of you may have had some initial success, only to get bored rather quickly and then find that you gained back the lost weight immediately after you stopped the diet. The reason is that losing weight is not only about calorie counting or restricting food intake; it is a holistic approach to how you live your life, from eating habits to your social life. Additionally, dieting rarely leads to permanent weight loss, and more importantly, a healthier lifestyle that is consistent; instead, it creates a feeling of helplessness and self-loathing, especially after you gain back the weight. These diet plans make you feel inadequate and a failure. The problem is that conventional diets do not tackle the underlying problem of weight loss and healthy living.

An underlying reason why most people are not successful in obtaining their goals when they are dieting is because the only thing, they are trying to change is their body – i.e., the outside, physical part. By doing this, you think you would feel happier and that your life would become much better. However, this is not always the case because what is really important, and to have true success, is what the SLOW Life diet uniquely incorporates: a different and changed mindset.

To change your mindset, though, requires sacrifice and dedication from you. The struggle is a constant factor, but real success to overcome this struggle comes from within. Sell yourself on what you are doing and trying to achieve; do it every day, feel it every day, live it every day. Over time, you will see a difference not only in the things you are doing, but also from the results of how you are doing them. You should aim to wake up every day with you convincing yourself that this is your day, and nothing will stop you from achieving what you want.

Instead of wasting time with another diet, I am going to show you the only truly effective method that works: creating a healthy lifestyle, the way the Greek villagers do. This notion encompasses all the problems you need to tackle to not only be healthier and lose weight properly, but also to make you feel better about yourself and to start appreciating who you truly are without having to compare yourself to your skinnier friend, your body-blessed neighbor, or the impossibly high standards of the supermodel you see in magazines. The beauty about creating a healthy lifestyle with the SLOW Life plan is that you do not need to rush; you are allowed to do it at your own pace. Of course, the more lackadaisical we are about making the change, the longer it will take - but that's fine. We are all different from one another, so find your ideal stride and run with it. Just like in the village where time is subjective to each and every resident! They take things at their own pace.

However, the one thing you must do is COMMIT TO IT for the long run because that is when you will truly see results. My aim is to help you create life-long sustainable habits that take no more energy than the habits you currently have, and that is what the SLOW Life diet is all about.

Table of Contents

LET'S GET STARTED

Let's dive in and get you familiarized with the changes you need to make to live the Greek village life that will create healthy habits, which you can simultaneously and immediately incorporate into your lifestyle.

Before going further, I should point out that the SLOW Life diet is based solely on research and experience of living in the Greek villages. This unique lifestyle and nutritional diet can most likely be found in many other parts of the Mediterranean, and thus may be similar to the aspects that the SLOW Life diet is founded on, but I cannot adhere to make any claims for these other parts. What I know is from my own experiences of living in a Greek village and adhering to that lifestyle.

As you read through this book, make sure to build up your reading according to the progression of the sections as they lead up to the chapter of implementing and incorporating the healthy habits found in the Greek villages. Look out for the tips throughout the various sections which will give you extra information or go into a little more detail for that specific idea/part, giving you a slightly more in-depth insight. Finally, pay close attention to the Challenges and Action Plans after each healthy habit because this will aid you with the changes to make in your lifestyle to put you on your way to that body you always wanted and happiness that has eluded you all these years.

Let's get started on the SLOW Life diet and begin living like a Greek villager!

Knowledge is Power

When you go through this book and study the challenges and action plan, always keep in mind that you will be educating yourself about your body and relating it to your daily routine and general lifestyle. These are the most important steps you can make towards your goals. This is because awareness and knowledge about fitness and nutrition are the most powerful tools you can have to take the first step.

TIP: Number one tip to lead a happier, more meaningful life, losing weight and increasing your life expectancy is to make small, realistic, achievable changes in your life with simple habits, which you can easily follow without tremendous suffering. Specifically, it is important for you to create healthy habits outlined in the SLOW Life diet not only to lose weight but to change your mindset and lifestyle for a healthier life.

What's great about the Greek village healthy, and socially-centric, habits are that they take little effort to incorporate in your own lives, as in one way or the other, you probably already incorporate some of them in your life right now without even having set foot in Greece or anywhere else in the region. These include having a healthy figure, feeling confident, having more energy, increasing your life expectancy, being happy by feeling happy, and by being surrounded by those you love and who love you back every single day. You're making these changes that will get you the results you seek without having to go through the pain and misery that a strict, calorie-counting diet puts on your body and your mental state.

We will embark on this journey together and we will reprogram your mindset. Do not think of this as a diet but rather a nutritional lifestyle. You will see the results will start to come when you mold your lifestyle and mindset to have these positive habits as the norm, practicing them every day and having them become second nature to you. This is the essence of the SLOW Life diet.

I. Greek Village lifestyle: Why does it work?

Although it would be tempting to jump right in and get to the action plan for implementing changes into your lifestyle, it would be beneficial to give you little context of why the basis of the SLOW Life diet is something that has been gaining notoriety in recent years. Being Greek and a third-generation olive oil producer, I have grown up with many of the Greek village lifestyle elements incorporated into my life, especially the eating habits. This is how most Greeks were raised and lived their life. It is part of the upbringing, lifestyle, and culture.

A major part of a village life is to turn down the chaotic rhythms of life. Slow life in a village goes hand in hand with having a simplified lifestyle where you can practice self-care. Greeks do not freak out if something has to be postponed or if plans get cancelled – the lifestyle is very much about going with the flow and mindful slowness, quality over quantity. The abundantly used phrase of *siga-siga*, which means *slowly-slowly*, gives merit to the way a Greek lives, especially in the villages. Metaphorically, though, it means to take a deep breath, to embrace the moment you are in, to practice self-caring, and to then…exhale.

The Slow Life diet is all about lifestyle. It is a road that leads to health, good habits, and happiness. It is a condition according to which the soul lives calmly and steadily, being disturbed by nothing. It focuses on eating right and creating healthy life habits. Greek villagers live their life in a way that focus on their lifestyle and their habits.

However, it was only in the 1950s that these eating habits and the effects they had started to be investigated and really studied and seen in a different light. As we have evolved and understood more about these eating habits, it was revealed that they are more of a way of life rather than just about consuming food for the sake of consuming and losing weight.

There is no doubt that your lifestyle dictates how you live, and that lifestyle is an important factor of health. According to the World Health Organization (WHO), 60% of related factors to individual health and quality of life are correlated to lifestyle. [4] And we can see the quality of life that people have in Greece, and other parts of the Mediterranean, as the Greek village lifestyle is about incorporating exercise (albeit in a meaningful and purposeful way) and relaxing into your daily routine. Doing the gardening, visiting a friend at sunset when the day has quieted, going to a shop to do your daily tasks, or taking a brisk walk after dinner is common practice and usually done by your own devices. Some of my friends and family living on

---

[4] The WHO cross-national study of health behavior in school-aged children from 35 countries: findings from 2001-2002. J Sch Health, 2004 Aug: 74(6): 204-6

Lesvos, oftentimes go on an evening stroll along the boardwalk and beach road in Mytilene, the capital city, after dinner.

Another important factor in the lifestyle is that meals are not rushed. There is no habit of mindlessly eating your food in front of the computer and/or television and shoving it down as quickly as possible to save time. Eating at the table with no electronic device found anywhere near the "temple of food" is a way to relax with family and friends while enjoying the flavors and aromas of local fare. Lunch can be a 1 ½ to 2-hour event and in some areas, stores are even closed during this time, giving employees and owners time to enjoy lunch and even sneak in a nap before returning for their afternoon shift. This gives a glimpse into what the SLOW Life diet encapsulates.

II. Basis of SLOW Life diet

A good basis to start is with the traditional Mediterranean Diet Pyramid as this will set the parameters of the SLOW Life plan.

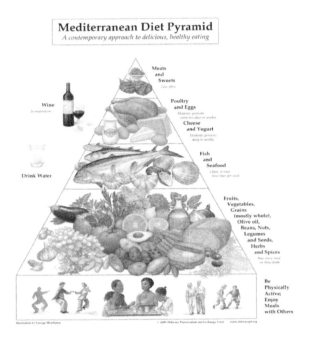

This pyramid was developed by Oldways Preservation Trust in 1993 and was based on studies made from the dietary patterns of the Mediterranean, specifically Greece and parts of Southern Italy, beginning in the 1960s. However, the interesting part of the new Pyramid is that it does not focus only on principal diet practices but also lifestyle practices, which actually play a vital role in the success of this pyramid. The largest part of the pyramid, the foundation, is devoted to the lifestyle practices people in the Mediterranean region follow. It is vital to engage in daily physical activity for good health, not only in planned activities such as aerobics and running, but also to incorporate it in our daily living, such as cleaning the house, taking the stairs instead of the elevator/escalator, and doing yard work. This is the key principle to the success of the diet and the structure of the pyramid.

In order to understand the working of the SLOW Life diet and what it entails for your nutrition and your lifestyle, let's look at the base of the pyramid first.

A. Bottom of Pyramid

One key message in the Pyramid is to engage in daily physical activity for good health. This includes planned activities like walking, dancing, and playing sports/games with others. However, the important part is not what you do, but it is rather on being physically active in daily living, as stated above.

In addition, the base of the Pyramid supports using foods as a means to pleasure and enjoyment. Eating and drinking in the company of others, savoring meals slowly, and sitting down at a meal can help achieve this.

We will get into more detail about this, but to touch up on it now, eating and drinking in the company of others tremendously boosts mental health and the pleasure of consuming what is in front you. The more often people eat with others, the more likely they are to feel happy and satisfied with their lives. Communal eating increases social bonding and feelings of well-being and enhances one's sense of contentedness and embedding within the community, including the familial community.

B. Second level

Fruits, Vegetables, Grains, Olive Oil, Beans, Nuts, Legumes, Seeds, Herbs and Spices

All these are central to a healthy diet, and that is why all of these foods fall into the same category, completing the entire base of the Mediterranean Diet Pyramid. These plant-based foods should be enjoyed at each and every meal, as research shows they promote heart health, overall health, and weight control.

We will go over these foods and level later on.

C. Third level

Fish and Seafood

An ever-growing body of research links fish consumption (an excellent source of essential fatty acids called Omega-3) to improved cardiovascular health and brain development and lower risk of chronic disease. What's more, when compared to beef, fish is a healthier lower-saturated fat protein source. Enjoy in at least two meals per week.

D. Fourth level

Poultry and Eggs, Yogurt and Cheese

Unlike the typical Western diet, poultry, eggs, yogurt and cheese are enjoyed less frequently throughout the week. Poultry and eggs are a good source of protein and can be consumed a few times per week. Be sure to remove skin from poultry and choose the white meat to reduce intake of saturated fat. As for eggs, if you have raised cholesterol, it is still fine to consume even three to four eggs per week because the cholesterol in eggs does not have a significant effect on blood cholesterol.[5] Dairy foods are consumed frequently but in moderate portions daily or weekly; the calcium in cheese and yogurt is important for bone and heart health. If you are worried about consuming higher portions of dairy products, you can choose 1% or non-fat milk, low-fat or non-fat yogurt to ease these

---

[5] If you have raised cholesterol, it's much more important to limit the amount of saturated fat you eat. Too much saturated fat can raise the cholesterol in your blood.

concerns. Good quality cheese should be limited to a few portions per week.

E. Tip of Pyramid

Red Meat and Sweets

Because red meat is not as readily available in Mediterranean regions, and producing it is costly (both financially and environmentally), as it is in the United States, it is consumed rather sparingly. Because of its higher saturated fat content, beef and pork should be limited, portion sizes controlled, and only lean cuts chosen when you do consume them.

Where dessert is concerned, its high sugar and fat content (and little to no nutrient value) relegates it to the "less often" recommendation for consumption. Fresh fruits, as a substitute for quenching sugar cravings, are great in taste, lower in calories, and have a much better nutrient profile.

III. The Secret Behind the SLOW Life diet

As stated before, the secret behind the Village health plan is not really about dieting in the traditional sense, nor about losing weight and simply following an eating plan, but rather, it is about a changed mindset. It's a lifestyle that demands a mindset that is committed to change and growth. The complete SLOW Life diet is about gearing every aspect of your life towards getting your mental and physical health in tip-top shape.

But why is a mindset, a change in lifestyle, important for success? Because mindset plays a critical role in how you cope with life's challenges, including weight loss and your mental health. This whole process of pushing aside the bad habits to replace them with the habits that will make you feel happier, fulfilled, and aid you to live longer, helps you persist in your efforts.

It is a simple concept that if you have a positive outlook on life, you will probably be happier than someone who can't look on the bright side. If you set goals for yourself with an action plan to follow through, you will probably reach more of your goals than someone who doesn't. That is why your mindset can impact all aspects of your life, from goal setting to mood. And because mindset always grows, try learning new techniques in order to improve on any skills that will play an aiding role in making your lifestyle transition.

IV. Why Should We Care?

All of us have our own reasons for wanting to live a healthier lifestyle. Maybe it is because we have low self-esteem because of our weight issues, we have low mobility, we feel depressed about unachieved goals, we have too much stress in our life, constantly on the move and not having enough time to take a deep breath, allowing bad habits dictate our mood, or constantly obsessing about our weight on the scale. No matter the reason, there is always one issue that slowly boils up and finally reaches a tipping point; it is the wake-up call!

My story starts at the core: my two children, the loves of my life. This, combined with my health, created the perfect conditions for my wake-up call.

One sunny day, feeling good about myself and without a care in the world, I made my way to the clinic, for what was supposed to be a routine checkup. After completing all the necessary tests, the general practitioner suggested I see a cardiologist. I was stunned by the recommendation, as there was no prior indication nor any hint that I needed to have my heart looked at. I took his advice and booked an appointment for a heart checkup.

All this made me start to question myself. Was it my eating habits, my way of life? Had I strayed too much from the path and was I indulging myself in unhealthy food habits and lifestyle? After a nervous couple of days of waiting for the appointment, and then to acquiesce through all of the doctor's commands and tests once that day arrived, the results were final. The cardiologist sat me down and said that my heart looked fine that day. But, he continued in a solemn voice, if I were to continue on the same path as I was treading, the following year he could not guarantee that I would have the same results. In other words, he saw that my heart was being strained by the "unhealthy" lifestyle and diet I was adhering to. I was overweight at 102 kg, borderline obese by definition as per my height and age. My blood results also showed that I had over the normal amount of cholesterol, 32% body fat, and a high uric acid content. The scary truth was that I was 38 years old and had a family; I was too young to have to think about any type of heart or health issues! This was my wake-up call with the question, what can I do to change my lifestyle to lead a healthier and have a longer life, at the forefront of my mind.

As you can see previously in the Pyramid, there is little wonder why the Mediterranean diet and lifestyle lead to a longer and healthier life.

It is important to point out that the Mediterranean Diet Pyramid's guidelines are based on the diet and lifestyle practices of areas such as Crete, mainland Greece, and Southern Italy in the 1960s. Research from that time-period indicated that people in these areas had the lowest rates of chronic disease in the world and life expectancy was of the highest at that time. Even now, two of the five places in the world that have been identified as having the longest living people (*see Ikaria and the blue zones below*) are from the Mediterranean region. And although the pace of life is picking up, fast food options are becoming more readily available, and stress has found its way into many people's lives in Greece and the Greek villages. However, the Greek Village health plan is still widely practiced, resulting in a longer and healthier lifestyle and leading to a happy life.

Still not convinced? You only have to read the numerous studies that have taken place on this lifestyle and eating habits. A UCLA study on the new approach to treating Alzheimer's disease[6] talks about just that. What the study revealed was that every participant demonstrated such marked improvement that almost all were found to be in the normal range on testing for memory and cognition by the study's end. In essence, this amounts to a cure. What's the catch? The results from this study were not due to an incredible new drug or medical breakthrough. The researchers used a protocol consisting of a variety of different lifestyle modifications to optimize metabolic parameters.[7] Specifically, participants were counseled to change their diet (eat a lot of veggies), exercise, develop techniques for stress management, and improve their sleep, among other interventions. In other words, the researchers opted to try changing the study group's

---

[6] *Reversal of Cognitive Decline in Alzheimer's* disease, https://www.aging-us.com/article/100981/text
[7] Ibid.

lifestyle and eating habits to see how it would affect their condition.   As stated above, the results were nothing more than remarkable.

V. The Centa...What?

If you have never heard of the Centenarians, or even the phrase "Blue Zones",[8] it refers to a study organized by scientists, and supported by the National Geographic Society, on the places where people live the longest, specifically, those who live to be 100 years old (i.e. cent). The term *blue zone* was coined by Dan Buettner.[9] The reason why it is called a *blue zone* is because the scientists who identified the first location – in Sardinia – drew a boundary in blue ink on a map, hence the term. An article in the *NY Times Magazine*.[10] described the blue zones as places "where people forget to die". Buettner contends that the kind of environment that defines a blue zone, which is a bit insulated from the comforts of modern life, is conducive to a hardiness and resilience that keeps the effects of aging at bay.[11]

In this study, there are five blue zones identified: Sardinia, Italy; Costa Rica; California; Japan, and

---

[8] *"Blue Zones" Where the World's Healthiest People Live*, https://www.nationalgeographic.com/books/features/5-blue-zones-where-the-worlds-healthiest-people-live/

[9] Buettner, Dan. *The Blue Zones Solution.* National Geographic Society, 2015.

[10] *The Island Where People Forget to Die,* https://www.nytimes.com/2012/10/28/magazine/the-island-where-people-forget-to-die.html

[11] The Blue Zones Solutions, ibid.

Ikaria, Greece. As you can see, two of the five are in the Mediterranean region.

Imagine a place so pristine and pure that the inhabitants often live more than a century without experiencing disease. Envisage an island where the pace of life is so stress-free that people who go there find themselves cured of illnesses and restored to health. This place is Ikaria, the last one on the list above, and it truly exists.

Ikaria is a small island in the Aegean Sea, southwest of the larger island Samos. According to tradition, it derives its name from Icarus, the son of Daedalus in Greek mythology, who was believed to have fallen into the sea nearby the island. Unlike Icarus, who died too young by flying too close to the sun and his wax wings melted causing him to plummet to the sea below, the residents of Ikaria are known to be part of the centenarian club (those who live to be 100). After the initial study, and even to present day, the Ikarians are known to have much lower rates of cancer and heart disease, suffer significantly less depression and dementia, maintain a sex life into old age and remain physically active deep into their 90s. Sound too good to be true? Well, it's not and Ikarians are living proof of this.

What is interesting from this study, and closely looking at the Ikarians, is that in their daily routine, they enforce the true "Greek lifestyle" - a combination of exercise and a quiet, stress-free life, suggesting that these are the secrets to a long and healthy lifestyle.

Ikaria is just a microcosm of what it is like in a Greek village that does not have the influence of modern life overtaking everyone's direction of life. They use technology as an aid to help themselves to better the community. And just like the residents in Ikaria, my own grandmother lived to be 92 years old, living all her life in the picturesque village of Agia Paraskevi on the island of Lesvos. She led a "blue zone" life that was natural to her because that was how she was brought up and lived. It not only revolved around a routine developed by her environment, but also from traditions

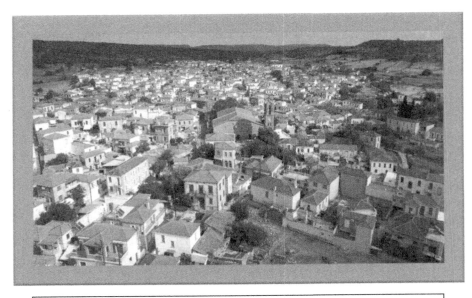

Ariel view of Agia Paraskevi on the island of Lesvos, Greece.

© Stratis Makrodoulis

and beliefs held strongly in her family. It was programmed in her as a part of her daily schedule and routine; in other words, it was her lifestyle.

I was able to get a first-hand look into this way of life. Growing up in the United States, my mother made it her duty to take me and my siblings to her roots. Every summer holiday, without fail. Don't get me wrong, it was a nice way to spend your summer, but as a child, you do not realize the significance of the wider picture. All you know is that you are away from your friends and spending your vacation in a place that is relatively foreign to you, and you have to adapt to that place you are in. What is interesting is that the memories you have as a grown-up are not only about the sights and sounds of the village and a time that is long past, like the cicadas chirping in the hot sun in the afternoon or the church bell tower chiming every hour breaking the silence of the afternoon siesta, but what comes rushing back are the things that have stuck with you from the way of life of these Greek villagers. They became so ingrained that I am now teaching them to my own children.

What I witnessed in my grandmother was that her daily routine consisted of waking up early, usually at sunrise. All those years that we would stay at her house, I never saw an alarm anywhere in the house – her internal clock would tell her when it was time to get up.

LIFESTYLE TIP: The University of Munich's Institute of Medical Psychology published a study that concludes that one overlooked culprit in the world's obesity epidemic may be the alarm clock. More specifically, the study explains our circadian clock must be rewound every day to keep it operating on a cycle of roughly 24 hours. It is reset by sunlight and darkness, the signals traveling to the brain through the optic nerve, and this natural system is disrupted by the alarm clock.[12] Try to "tune" your body by winding down with the sunset and letting the sunrise gently wake you, as opposed to the rude awakenings brought on by the alarm clock.

The routines that she programmed for herself, that suited her schedule and pace of life, would start by preparing herself for the tasks of the day, subsequently eating a light breakfast, usually consisting of lightly warm goat's milk with a piece of whole-wheat *paksimadi* (dry rusk), and honey obtained from local producers, spread on the rusk. Other times, she would eat local yogurt made from pasteurized milk (goat or cow) accompanied by oats. In the summertime, fresh, seasonal fruit was eaten with the yogurt.

After breakfast, she would tend to her garden, full of blossoming flowers and plants, which she knew by

---

[12] *Your Alarm Clock May be Hazardous to your Health,* https://www.smithsonianmag.com/science-nature/your-alarm-clock-may-be-hazardous-to-your-health-164620290/

name and blossoming season. This was her pride and joy, her eyes lighting up every time she would tend to these plants and flowers as if she was entering them in a floral competition every single day. She watered, pruned, and tilled the soil. Simultaneously, she would clean and organize the yard. This task of gardening was her passion, and she gave time to it every day, as it gave her enjoyment and pleasure. However, at the same time she was doing something joyous which consisted of being outdoors, she was also partaking in physical activity. Nothing else seemed to matter; the experience was so enjoyable that she did it for the sheer sake of doing it. She would experience happiness in its purest form.

Following this, she would start preparing the lunch menu. This usually was paired with a walk to the village center to do her daily shopping, mostly the food that would be cooked that day for lunch and/or dinner. The stops usually included the bakery, the butcher, the convenient store, and the delicatessen. While visiting these shops - which were owned by the friends she had grown up with - she would also run into neighbors and other friends, all of whom would be doing their daily chores at that time as well. An important point to note here is that this was not only a time to do the daily and weekly shopping, but it was also a time to get up to speed with the village news; a sort of social newspaper if you will. She would then return home from her errand-run in the village and prepare lunch, subsequently doing house chores, and any other task that needed to be tended to and as time permitted.

One thing I noticed is that she never exerted stress upon herself if she could not get something done, and she never pushed back her schedule to finish that something. If it was done within the time frame allowed, great. If she could not finish, then she would put it aside and do it at the next available slot in her schedule. However, what I observed was a remarkable trait of always being organized; she prioritized the important things, something we can all learn as a life skill.

After lunch, at around 1:00-2:00 p.m., it would be nap time - mandatory in the summertime - and this would be for about 1-1.5 hours long. After waking from the nap and having a healthy snack, usually consisting of either yogurt, nuts, or fruit, friends would come over in the afternoon and sit on the patio near her prized and luscious garden, under the aromatic azalea plant, and just talk, about the happenings of the day and other life matters that occupied them at the time.

At dusk, either she would go to afternoon church service or if she stayed at home, the neighbors would gather to talk outside in the neighborhood *plateia* (central square), where the kids would play and grown-ups would discuss different matters, sing, and reminisce about old times. This was called the *yeitonia*, which is literally, the neighborhood.

It has been studied that close friendships provide a buffer for stressful living that is likely to play out through your immune and endocrine systems, allowing you to age healthier. Having strong connections is just as important for health as exercise. An ongoing study that began in 1976, revealed that among the oldest women, those who didn't have at least one confidante showed the same decline in physical functioning and vitality as heavy smokers and the most severely overweight. Conversely, the more quality friends a woman had, the better shape she was in.

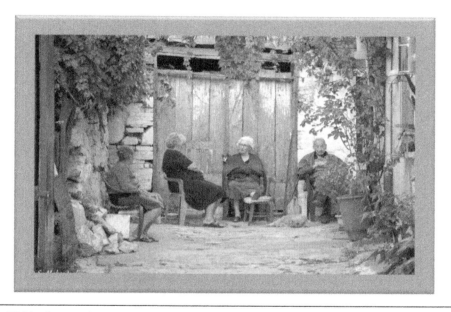

Old ladies and man sitting outside in the 'yeitonia' at dusk to chat in a calm environment. This was in the village of Agiassos on the island of Lesvos.

This routine is a snapshot, yet typical, of a Greek villager living a simple life. My grandmother was surrounded by the things she loved, physical activity was incorporated in her daily routine through her passion, friends and family were always close by, and her faith was a big part of her life.

The reason I wanted to describe her routine in such an organized and fairly detailed manner is not because I am asking you to mimic her schedule, or the schedule of the people in Ikaria, but instead, to take the elements that make up this particular lifestyle and see what all these Greek people have in common and to try to incorporate these aspects into your own lives, wherever you live in the world. Specifically, my grandmother encapsulated all these factors that she structured as part of her life and gave her purpose and made her a valuable part of society. This is the power of this type of lifestyle: it gives you a sense of direction and meaning without always searching for and wanting more.

Let's look back at my grandmother's routine and see what common threads we notice. Firstly, food was an important part of her daily routine. Traditional diet included lots of vegetables and olive oil, limited amounts of dairy and meat products, and moderate alcohol. However, there was always an emphasis on potatoes, goat's milk, honey, legumes (lentils and garbanzo), wild greens, fruit, and some fish. Cheese and yogurt were consumed to fulfil the daily dairy requirements.

An important point that we should take into account is that red meat and poultry were consumed only one time a week - two if you there was a special occasion. Fish was the preferred "meat" and eaten twice a week. Sweets were rarely consumed during the week but perhaps, again, on special occasions, but normally, they were eaten only about two times per week. Remember though, honey was consumed in tea, in the morning as a spread, or with yogurt which fulfilled the sweet cravings, with the upside of not having put on empty calories as you do with eating sugary sweets and simultaneously benefitting from the nutritional elements that honey offers.

This is what you would typically see all around Greek households. More importantly, you also see elements of this in kindergartens and schools. The weekly menu at a school (if food is cooked on site) is tailored around this nutritional diet, which goes to building the foundation of good habits. This is crucial to establishing a routine of this lifestyle from an early age, as kids adopt this, and it becomes second nature to them.

Having a rest

Apart from her nutrition, we also saw an emphasis on her social activity and resting in the afternoon.

When foreigners go to visit Greece during the late spring and summer months, especially outside the main cities, they usually stumble across a rather strange site – shops and other commercial establishments being closed during the middle of the day and few people out and about. After playing detective and investigating the incident further, they tend to find out that these shops are on what is called a summer time schedule. Usually, the schedule is that the shops are open from 9 a.m. to about 2 p.m., they then close for a couple of hours and reopen from 5 p.m. until about 9 p.m. The first reaction to this is "how lazy are these people!" However, there is a more valid reason for this schedule and it does not have to do with laziness.

The simple answer is that the people are napping. Yes, napping! Due to the extreme heat during the summer months, people close the shop during the hottest part of the day and open-up during the most bearable times. Additionally, as the summer day was longer, splitting the day into two would allow people to function throughout the day with less stress and more energy. Therefore, the reason behind napping is for health and had nothing to do with the work integrity of the nation.

The other interesting thing about her schedule, and what I noticed while growing up, was that all activities, even shopping, involved a social interaction and exercise since everything was local and in close proximity. This meant that the preferred mode of transport was walking and because people knew each other and socialized, the activity became more enjoyable rather than being a boring chore, not just to yourself, but to everyone who crossed paths with you.

Additionally, my grandmother's neighbors were her best friends, as they not only grew up together, but they also shared the same values as her and helped each other out when needed. She was a regular church goer with a strong faith, and she regularly involved herself in church activities.   This included charity work, excursions, and community gatherings.   Throughout the year, but especially in the summer where she could sit outside until dusk, the daily meet up in the afternoon was with her friends in the neighborhood or at someone's yard, and they would just talk for hours, about life, activities, religion, family, knitting, cooking, and anything else that would interest them.

V. Putting It into Practice

After reading the above chapters, most of it may still look foreign to you in a literal and practical sense, and no doubt many of you have one question in mind: How do I implement, let alone successfully implement, this CHANGE in my life? Yes, this change, because that is exactly what we are aiming to achieve. We are striving to change the part of your lifestyle that has not produced positive results...yet. The more you feed your negative habits, the more your lifestyle will be dictated by these. As a result, the negative thoughts start to seep in while low self-esteem and lethargy become the norm. Staying within the confines of all this negative comfort is easy, and tempting, yet this is what creates an unhealthy lifestyle and mental state.

One statement I hear all the time is that it is easier to implement these habits when you live in Greece or another part of the Mediterranean because all these things are accessible and ingrained in society. Generally, this is true as it is easier to do something when your environment dictates it and where it surrounds you. You tend to follow the rules of the society in which you live, and which are most likely not aligned with the Greek lifestyle. However, always keep this in mind: it is not about becoming Greek or replicating Greece's societal infrastructure and norms; it is more about adopting these village habits and incorporating them into your life the way you see fit.

First and foremost, you must take baby steps and keep things simple. Don't overwhelm yourself with implementing all the habits at once. These habits, in essence, are not difficult and not foreign to most, and as an added bonus, a lot of them already exist in your daily routine. Before you know it, you will have more habits integrated in your lifestyle than you realize.

Remember, although it is advised to take small steps in your journey, in order to truly make positive changes occur, you need to overcome the status quo of your current lifestyle and incorporate these changes because they are crucial to the success of reaching your goals.

Therefore, let's start breaking down the stages in your quest and individually study the habits that you will need to implement, step-by-step and in a fun and easy way, so you can achieve success the Greek village way.

TIP: To get you started on your journey, receive a complimentary 1-week menu that is based on the Greek village lifestyle and very nutritional. Scan the QR code at the end of the book to get it in your inbox for free.

The Village 12: Unique Habits

The Village lifestyle diet can be broken down into 12 important health-related categories. Things will be laid out in the following format: listing each health habit, some information of its importance, and a challenge for the best way to implement it into your lifestyle. Look out also for some Tips, throughout this list, where important information will be given for clarification or just as extra options to aid you in your goal.

1. Village Habit 1: Make it a Social Experiment!

The Greeks knew something that scientists are just discovering now. The simple act of being social brings about positive emotional and physical health benefits. Psychologists and scientists have conducted studies that reveal that simply talking to a friend or loved one at the dinner table can play a big role in relieving stress and boosting mood. Eating with others can also prevent overeating, making it as healthy for your waistline as it is for your outlook. It is known that communal eating not only activates beneficial neurochemicals but also improves digestion. The dining table provides an opportunity for conversation, storytelling, and reconnection. When you bond with others and experience a sense of connection, it leads to well-being and contentedness,[13] thus preventing you from gorging. Switch off the tv and computer, put away and hide your smartphone, and connect to someone real over a meal!

My fondest memories in my yiayia's house were around the lunch table. Usually, we would spend the morning out of the house, either going to the local beach with friends, doing some chores or running errands. We knew that at 1-2 pm, when it was lunchtime, we would come back to the house and the table was perfectly set, with a knitted, white table cloth handmade by my yiayia displaying an intricate set of patterns, the everyday chinaware with cutlery laid out, and always a napkin folded perfectly under the fork. We all had our favorite spots to sit, and we all would sit down as my yiayia and mother would bring out the always aromatic and delicious meal to be served. All of us would enjoy savoring not only the food prepared but also being all together, talking about the day's events and any other topic that we felt was worth talking about.

Meals are not rushed, nor are they eaten in front of an electronic device and shoved down as quickly as possible. They are never consumed on the go, in the car, or speed walking between "important" meetings (sound familiar?). It's a way to relax with family and friends while enjoying the flavors and aromas of the

---

[13]   "Mealtimes   and   Mental   Health". https://www.mentalhealth.org.uk/a-to-z/m/mealtimes-and-mental-health

local fare. They just enjoy living in the moment. As family plays a hugely important part in Greeks', and other Mediterraneans', lives, family meals are also made into a regular occurrence. Meals not only provide comfort to everyone, including kids, but they are a great way to catch-up and monitor eating habits as well.

Another way to practice this act of slowing down and sitting down is called mindful eating. Mindful eating is about allowing yourself to become aware of the positive and nurturing opportunities that are available through food selection and preparation by respecting your inner wisdom. It also practices using all of your senses in choosing to eat food that is both satisfying to you and nourishing to your body. Along with acknowledging responses to food, you become aware of physical hunger and satiety cues to guide your decisions to begin and end eating.

The benefits of mindful eating are that it can reduce physiological distress such as depression, anxiety, stress, and eating behaviors including binge eating. Mindful eating can also result in weight loss for overweight and obese people. And this is because it provides a way to improve the body's natural ability to control an eating behavior.

What most of us are doing now is the complete opposite. Instead of mindful eating, we engage in *mindless* eating. We are eating food with thousands of calories not because we are hungrier, but because it is just there. We have never lived in a time in our human history of such abundance and accessibility to food than we do now. And because it is so readily and easily accessible on every corner, the result is that when we are eating, we do so without realizing that we are eating. And because we are not focused on what we eat, we tend to eat unhealthy food that does not make us full whilst we are distracted. In a recent study, it was found that people ate more whilst watching TV than in any of the other situations looked at in the study, and the amount people ate whilst driving was unrelated to changes in their hunger. This indicates that we eat more when we are distracted, particularly when watching TV.[14]

As shown earlier, the Med Pyramid placed this part of being social in every aspect of your life at the bottom as this is the foundation and the most important part of making your lifestyle change. It not only prevents us from eating mindlessly while being distracted by insignificant things like TV and driving, but being social and socially eating is the key to not only making a physical change, but also the mental change that is necessary to give you balance and ultimate success in your goal.

The Greek villagers use food as a means to pleasure and enjoyment. Eating and drinking in the company of others, savoring meals slowly, and sitting down at a meal are all common things that come from the respecting and enjoying the food and having a lifestyle

---

[14] Wansink, B., *Mindless eating: Why we eat more than we think.* 2nd edition (2009) London: Hay House.

that slows life down is a part of the culture that is ingrained in each person of the village. The food becomes a gateway to a healthy life and happiness that can only be observed in the Greek villages.

TIP: Wanting to expand your social network? Share meal with others to achieve social notoriety. If you live alone, cook a little extra and invite a friend, co-worker, or neighbor to join you. Or, look for groups that share the same interests with you and go out once a week for dinner together! This will also be a good test as to how you are able to maintain your nutritional habits when ordering from a restaurant.

TIP #2: Four hands are better than two. Invite a friend to share shopping and cooking for a Greek or Mediterranean meal. Cooking, not only eating, with others can be a fun way to deepen relationships, and splitting the costs can make it cheaper for both of you.

a. Activities

We, as human beings, are social animals who remain group-oriented to ensure survival, connection, and belonging. Our lives begin in family groups, and we function thereafter as members of groups at school, work, and in communities. The origin of the power of the group as an agent of change to promote healing lies buried in antiquity. Thus, it is no exception that doing things in groups, like exercising, boosts your mental state and increases your probability of achieving your goal.

And this concept is anything other than foreign to Greek villagers. In my village, there is a religious festival of the Tavros (bull), honoring *Aghios* (Saint) Haralambos. It happens every July and combines a variety of happenings, including eating, drinking, dancing, a horse procession on the main street of the village all decorated with colorful and elaborate accessories, horse races, and church services, all in connection to the ritual of the bull's sacrifice. It is one of the biggest happenings in the village's calendar.

At a designated place in the village, a large black cauldron, worn and charred by its many years of service, stands sturdy on a crackling, fire pit. The men tend to the fire, while the women assemble all the ingredients needed to make the traditional and local *kisketch* dish. These include chopped onions, wheat, bull's meat and fat mixed with olive oil. The large cauldron is filled with fresh spring water to the brim. Then the ingredients are added one by one. The meal took 5-6 hours to cook.

In the meantime, traditional music would be playing from an old FM radio, one with the knobs to turn the analog needle. There would be some dancing and wine drinking, the women huddling around the cauldron talking about daily happenings, while the children would play hide-and-seek, tag, or any other games they conjured up in the nearby square. People would flow by like leaves on a stream, stopping to have a chat or a drink, and then continuing on their way, taking a stroll to the center square.

As the sun would set and the time drew nearer to the end of the boil, with the buttery aroma wafting through the evening air, the people gather around the cauldron and the *kisketch* is communally served for the whole village to enjoy. We would take several steaming containers back home, and for neighbors who were too elderly and could not make, someone would always make sure that they would get a portion of the village meal as well, never to be left out of this time-honoured tradition.

These communal activities are important to village life. The reason why this type of activity results in an increase in mental well-being, is because it brings the community together for a common goal, a common cause which they can share together. This in turn translates to more successes as individuals and as a community. Subsequently, community involvement provides a sense of belonging and social connectedness. Having people to talk to and depend on and making new connections through hobbies or a social group, can be extremely helpful.

2. Village Habit 2: Greens Galore

This heading is not hard to understand. As you probably have heard many times before, you can't go wrong by eating too many vegetables!

One of the things the Mediterranean diet emphasizes is eating primarily plant-based foods. An abundance and variety of plant foods should make up the majority of your meals. You should be striving to eat approximately 5-7 servings of vegetables a day.

The reason why vegetables are an important part of the Med diet and major part of the Mediterranean's lifestyle is because eating a variety of colorful vegetables is a sure-fire way to reap the array of nutrients and antioxidants these plant foods offer.

One of the main health benefits of vegetables is their high nutrient content. Vegetables are loaded with vitamins and minerals that contribute to growth and the maintenance of good health. For example, vegetables are high in potassium, which is important for healthy blood pressure. Various vitamins, such as C and A, help keep eyes, skin, teeth and gums healthy, fight infection, and promote wound healing. Perhaps most importantly, vegetables are rich in a particular group of nutrients called antioxidants, which fight cellular damage and help prevent heart disease, cancer, Parkinson's disease, atherosclerosis, heart attack, and Alzheimer's disease.

An abundant source of vegetables in Greece are wild "*horta*", or mountain greens/weeds. These are the dark horse of vegetables in Greece as they are easily accessible, and extremely healthy as they are considered to be a superfood. These wild greens pack a punch as they are extremely high in antioxidants, with a study indicating that they contain more antioxidants than blueberries.

These are a good source of iron, magnesium, potassium, and calcium, as well as carotenoids – colorful pigments the body converts to Vitamin A. Recent studies have recorded that a diet rich in nitrates from wild greens can also lower blood pressure and reduce the risk of glaucoma. They are also very good for your heart. Each area has some sort of locally grown greens, so research your area, find them, and dig in!

Wild greens are super easy to cook and garnishing them for flavor can be fun. The health benefits of this superfood really are second to none and they can be served as a side dish or as a meal with some protein. All you need to do is boil your greens, add a pinch of salt, drizzle with good Greek olive oil (preferably evo3 olive oil!) and lemon and you are ready to serve this simple, and ever-so-healthy dish.

TIP: Although it may sound difficult to find mountain greens, there are many greens to choose from. Try the following: spinach, collard greens, mustard greens, beet greens, kale, chicory, wilds such as dandelion, purslane, lamb's quarter, beetroot leaves and amaranth. Beetroot leaves and amaranth are personal favorites, and the good thing about beetroot leaves is that you can find them everywhere. These wild greens should be present at every lunch and dinner, minimum of one but aim for two servings per meal.

TIP #2: When searching for the right veggies, don't fret, they are easier to find than you think! As with fruits (listed later), Greeks eat their veggies with the seasons. To find seasonal veggies, visit your local farmers' market and sign up for your local CSA (Community Supported Agriculture). Try these to get you started, which should be easy to find locally grown: artichokes, dandelion greens, tomatoes, cucumbers, zucchini, eggplant, cabbage, and leeks. Along with the health benefits derived, eating vegetables can also make weight management easier. Most produce is low in calories compared to other types of food, so filling up on these foods can aid in weight loss, or, at the very least, help maintain your weight.

Vegetables also work as excellent substitutes in different recipes. For example, use fresh applesauce instead of butter or processed vegetable oil in muffins or cookies. Add sautéed vegetables to an omelet to make it more filling without a lot of calories. Or make cauliflower pizza dough for a healthy alternative.

CHALLENGE: Why not start a meal with a salad? This will fill you up with a healthy starter and consequently will prep you to eat less for the main course. Be careful though! Do not add fattening dressings to your salad – a hearty vinaigrette-extra virgin olive oil, or lemon dressing will give a fresh and full flavor.

CHALLENGE #2: When you have a craving for chips, pretzels, crackers and ranch dip, instead reach for carrots, celery, broccoli, and low-calorie salsa. These are viable and healthy alternatives!

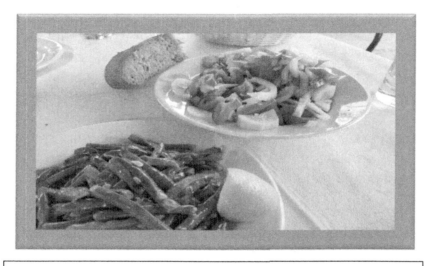

Typical dishes to have accompany a meal either at home or at a taverna. Greek salad drizzled in olive oil and boiled green beans with olive oil and lemon

3. Village Habit 3: Keep Your Virginity

Extra virgin olive oil is one of the healthiest fats, if not the most, that exists. This oil, a large part of the SLOW

Life diet and lifestyle, is a traditional fat that has been a dietary staple for some of the world's healthiest populations.

Before delving into why it is an important food to incorporate into your daily routine and lifestyle, you must understand the elements that make this food so healthy. As an olive oil producer who is reviving an age-old family tradition, I want to transfer my love and knowledge for this so called "liquid gold".

There are a wide variety of olive oils, all differing in their prices, for a consumer to choose from. Amidst all the different labels and brands, choosing which olive oil is best suited to your needs and tastes can be an overwhelming task. Nevertheless, with a little knowledge, you will be rightfully equipped next time you go shopping for your olive oil.

So, what are the different categories of olive oil? The following designations are the grades of oil extracted from the olive:

- **Extra Virgin**: The best/superior quality of olive oil available is described as "extra virgin" and produced solely by mechanical means. Extra virgin is the highest quality and most flavorful olive oil classification. In chemical terms it is described as having a free acidity, expressed as oleic acid, of not more than 0.8 grams/100 grams and a peroxide value of less than 20 milliequivalent O2. It must be produced entirely by mechanical means without the use of any solvents.

- **Virgin olive oil**: Olive oils described as "virgin" are those that have been obtained from the original fruit without having been synthetically treated and obtained directly by mechanical means. Once the olives have been picked, pressed, and washed, no other process has taken place other than decantation, and centrifugation to extract the oil, and filtration, and is usually up to 1.0 grams/100 grams of free acidity.
- **Olive oil**: Olive oil is the pure oil obtained from the fruit of olive trees. No oil obtained using solvents, re-esterification processes, or mixed with other vegetable oils qualifies under this description and is usually above the level of 1.0 grams/100 grams of free acidity.
- **Refined olive oil**: This is the olive oil obtained from virgin olive oils by refining methods which do not lead to alterations in the initial glyceride structure.
- **Olive-pomace oil**: oil comprising exclusively of oils obtained by treating the product obtained after the extraction of olive oil and oils obtained directly from olives.

TIP: **Organic extra virgin**: Although this is not a grade/classification, it is a testament to the way the olive groves were kept, and olives were harvested with sustainable practices in mind. Some say that organic extra virgin olive oil contains all the vitamins and nutrients of the olive fruit, and if you get a premium organic extra virgin olive oil, it will taste better and have a full aroma.

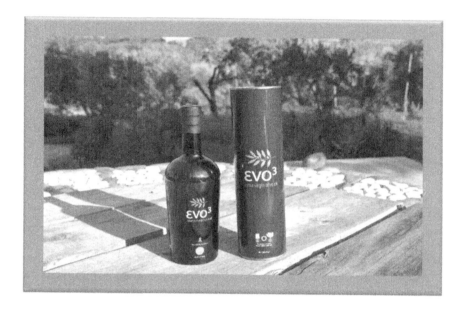

Evo3 extra virgin organic olive oil in the family groves on the island of Lesvos in Greece.

Why is extra virgin olive oil the healthiest? It contains modest amounts of Vitamins E and K and plenty of beneficial fatty acids. However, where extra virgin olive oil *really* shines is in its content of antioxidants. Some of the main antioxidants are the anti-inflammatory oleocanthal, as well as oleuropein, a substance that protects LDL cholesterol from oxidation.

There have also been numerous studies and research for the extensive health benefits that extra virgin olive oil can have. Many observational studies show that death from cardiovascular diseases is low in certain areas of the world, especially the countries around the Mediterranean Sea.

It has been shown that it can help prevent heart disease. In one major study, it reduced heart attacks, strokes, and death by 30%.

It has also been speculated that one of the mechanisms behind olive oil's benefits is its ability to fight inflammation. There is some evidence that oleic acid itself, the most prominent fatty acid in olive oil, can reduce inflammatory markers. Chronic inflammation can cause diseases such as heart disease, cancer, metabolic syndrome, diabetes, Alzheimer's, and arthritis.

Following this, studies have shown that people in Mediterranean countries have a fairly low risk of cancer which could be from compounds found in olive oil, i.e., oleic acid, which fights cancer on a molecular level.

The preliminary evidence of extra virgin olive oil is that it can fight Alzheimer's disease. One feature of Alzheimer's is a buildup of protein tangles called beta amyloid plaques, in certain neurons in the brain. A study in mice showed that a substance in olive oil can help to clear these plaques from the brain. A human controlled trial showed that a Mediterranean Diet enriched with olive oil had favorable effects on brain function and reduced the risk of cognitive impairment.

I have heard many people say, and you may have read many stories online, that cooking with olive oil is unhealthy and that it will degrade the oil, thus, making it dangerous to eat. Even George Mateljan, chef and author of *The World's Healthiest Foods* book, has a specific section on his website about why he does not cook with olive oil.

However, all this information that is being written about not cooking with olive oil is misguided and the only thing that one has to do to put this to rest is look at the heating point of olive oil.

The first argument that these pundits make is that olive oil loses its color and all its nutrients when fried. The second argument is that due to a low smoke point, it would turn the healthy fat into a smoky, stinky, free-radical-releasing mess when heated, and would make it rancid – a state that declassifies extra virgin olive oil to a lower-grade (lampante) olive oil.

The first argument has been touted by supporters of not using extra virgin olive oil for cooking ever since olive oil has been deemed a "good" fat. However, this opinion is a myth. Firstly, heart-healthy mono-unsaturated fats are not unfavorably altered by heat. They survive a sauté intact. Now, research is showing that other plant-based compounds—the elements that likely give olive oils their complex flavor profiles as well as other healthful properties—can also stand up to standard cooking procedures. They're surprisingly stable, as long as the oil is not heated past its smoking point, which for extra-virgin olive oil is pretty high—about 405°F or 210°C.

The smoking point, which makes the olive oil stable, is also the main point concerning the second argument. What is the smoke point? It is the temperature at which oil will start to smoke when heated. So, can cooking with olive oil make it a free-radical mess? The answer is no. Olive oil is four to five times more resistant to heat than seed oils or butter, and it can be heated until 405°F or 210C without smoking. The fact is that the average cooktop heats to between for high heat setting 300° and 500°F (150 - 260°C). So, unless you go above this point of 405°F or 210C, which is quite high for a household anyway as we have to be cautious of cooking at such high temperatures, then this argument becomes debunked.

Additionally, experts say that olive oil is one of the most stable vegetable oils under cooking/heating conditions. The reason is that fatty acids composition (mostly formed by monounsaturated fat), allow olive oil to be more resistant than other oils, since it is significantly

64

less unsaturated than the majority of other vegetable oils.[15]

TIP: Even though extra virgin olive oil has a lower smoke point than regular olive oil -- that doesn't mean you shouldn't cook with it either. Just keep your burner down if you don't want your olive oil or extra virgin olive oil to reach its smoke point. As said above, the average stovetop is between 200 to 300°F (95 - 150°C) on medium/low heat, so try to aim for the lower end of that range, especially if you're cooking with extra virgin.

CHALLENGE: Eat more of this monosaturated fat. Research findings are clear that it is very important to decrease the use of highly saturated fats like butter, lard, shortening, palm kernel oil, coconut oil, and any other oil that has been hydrogenated. Thus, try to use extra virgin olive oil as a healthy replacement for butter or margarine. Use it in cooking, marinating, and garnishing. Dip bread in flavored olive oil or lightly spread it on whole-grain bread for a tasty alternative to butter.

4. Village Habit 4: Cool Beans

---

[15] *Yes, Cooking With Olive Oil is Perfectly Safe,* Leigh Weingus. https://www.huffpost.com/entry/olive-oil-explainer_n_55b925cce4b0a13f9d1b5143?ncid=engmodushpmg00000004

Legumes are a low-fat, high-protein source of vitamins, minerals, antioxidant compounds, and dietary fiber. What does this mean? To put it simply, it means that legumes are nutrient-dense foods, or those that deliver a wide range of nutrients for relatively few calories, that provide energy and nourish your body and supports good health.

TIP: Examples of legumes are lentils, broad beans, kidney, fava, cranberry beans, navy beans, black beans, chickpeas, and yellow split peas.

The Mediterranean people love eating legumes. It is a stable part of their diet. The Greeks eat all kind of legumes, but their favorite, and the most common legumes that you find in their dishes are lentils, fava, chickpeas, and large kidney beans. Go to any taverna and you will find at least one, if not two of these legumes on every table!

But what is the big deal about legumes? Why do Greeks bother with them and why it is such a big part of the SLOW Life diet?

Well, the beauty about legumes is that they are high in antioxidant nutrients, dietary fiber, cholesterol-free, naturally low in fat, and plant/vegetable protein. What this translates into for losing weight is that legumes make you feel fuller longer and, therefore, help prevent the hunger that can lead to unhealthy snacking and unwanted pounds; what this also translates into for health is that evidence shows that consuming more plant-based foods lowers the risks of heart disease, high blood pressure, stroke, and type 2 diabetes.

To understand better how legumes, a fibrous food, positively affect weight management, we must look at how fiber affects the body. Fiber boosts satiety meaning its intake will make you feel full for hours. This way you can control further food intake to avoid overeating. Many dieticians recommend adding legume vegetables to weight loss diet programs because, aside from its satiety boosting effects, it also regulates digestion thus assures the removal of toxins and also the prevention of fat formation in the body.

Although the above helps us understand the result of eating legumes, it still does not answer why they feature heavily in the Village eating lifestyle. It is for the obvious facts that they are economically affordable and obtainable all year round. Few plant proteins that have such a boost to health in every sense can be found throughout the year.

TIP: What the Greeks say about legumes is enjoy them as the basis of meatless main dishes and you won't miss the animal protein!

TIP #2: The easiest way to increase your intake is by tossing a handful in soups or salads, or make your own veggie burgers by mixing beans, vegetables, breadcrumbs and egg whites to bind them together.

TIP #3: Gradually add them to your diet if you experience excess gas from eating beans and other legumes. This gives your digestive tract time to adjust to the extra fiber and helps prevent unwanted side effects.

CHALLENGE:
1) Why don't you prepare soups, stews and casseroles that feature legumes?

2) Use pureed beans as the basis for dips and spreads. Try various types of beans and find your favorite ones. Be creative!

3) Add chickpeas or black beans to salads. If you typically buy a salad at work and no beans are available, bring your own from home in a small container and just pop them on top. This way, you will be sure to get your dose of legumes.

4) Add cooked beans to meatballs or burgers.

5) Snack on a handful of legume nuts, e.g. soybean, peanuts, toasted chickpeas (in Greece they are called *stragalia*), rather than on chips or crackers.

6) Every week try to have one legume day in your weekly meal plan.

CHALLENGE #2: If you like eating white rice with stir-fried meat, why not try substituting it with the Village version of legumes and stir-fried vegetables. It's all about experimenting and being creative in the kitchen, and it will go a long way to getting you where you want to be.

---

5. Village Habit 5: Get Fruity and Nutty

Fruits

Fruit and nuts are commonly found in the Village recipes, so let's look at the benefits of each of these, starting with fruits, which are widely eaten and used.

Fresh fruits are abundant in the SLOW Life diet. We all know the various sayings and studies that fruits are good for you and that we should be eating more of them throughout the day, every day. However, why are they so healthy and why do the Greeks eat them in abundance?

The why is rather easy: eating fruit provides health benefits — people who eat more fruits and vegetables as part of an overall healthy diet are likely to have a reduced risk of some chronic diseases, such as reducing the risk of heart disease, including heart attack and stroke. They can also protect against certain types of cancers. Studies have also shown that a diet rich in fibrous foods may reduce obesity and type 2 diabetes. Fruits are lower in calories per cup instead of some other higher-calorie foods which is useful in helping lower caloric intake.

The reasoning behind the why is that fruits provide nutrients vital for health and maintenance of your body.

Most fruits are naturally low in fat, sodium, and calories. None have cholesterol.

There are also some fruits that are rich in a class of natural molecules called phytochemicals. In the body, these are usually involved in some stage of metabolism. On the opposite end, these molecules are also under intense study for their favorable effect on the skin, which contributes to the aesthetic effect of aging and living the natural life.

Fruits are also sources of many essential nutrients that are under-consumed, including potassium, dietary fiber, Vitamin C, and folate (folic acid). Dietary fiber is important for proper bowel function. It helps reduce constipation and diverticulosis. Fiber-containing foods such as fruits help provide a feeling of fullness with fewer calories, which goes a long way into losing weight.

TIP: Whole or cut-up fruits are sources of dietary fiber; fruit juices contain little or no fiber. Therefore, cut down on drinking fruit juices and opt-out for eating real fruit!

Vitamin C is important for growth and repair of all body tissues, helps heal cuts and wounds, and keeps teeth and gums healthy.

Folate (folic acid) helps the body form red blood cells. Women of childbearing age who may become pregnant should consume adequate folate from foods. This reduces the risk of neural tube defects, spina bifida, and anencephaly during fetal development.

As you can see, there is little doubt as to why Greeks eat so much fruit. But what is interesting as well is that Greeks associate fruits with seasons. In the summertime, fresh fruit becomes a way to hydrate, cool down in the sun, but most importantly, it is seen as a healthy way to indulge your sweet tooth. Instead of choosing ice cream or another desert that is readily available, because fruits are always found in the home, snacking on fruit becomes a first option rather than an alternative.

TIP: Keep fresh fruit visible at home and keep a piece or two at work so you have a healthful snack when your stomach starts growling. Lots of grocery stores stock exotic fruit—pick a new one to try each week and expand your fruit horizons. Even more so now, it is easy to find ready cut individual packages of fruits to avoid the hassle of cutting or cleaning fruits, so there is no excuse!

TIP #2: If it helps you to eat more, add a little sweetness to it - drizzle some honey over slices of pear or sprinkle a little brown sugar on grapefruit. However, fruits already have natural sugar in them: eat up so you won't crave that muffin or donut!

TIP #3: Aim to get one or two pieces of fruit per meal, or better yet, between meals. Fruit should be the most frequent dessert.

CHALLENGE: When choosing from the supermarket, buy fruits that are in season. Look for these when they are in season: figs, pomegranates, apricots, melons, apples, pears, lemons, and grapes. Also, to alternate and keep things interesting for your nutritional wellbeing, try opting for dry fruits as well. You can add both fresh and dried fruits to salads, Greek yogurt, or oatmeal as toppings.

Nuts are another component of a healthy SLOW Life diet. Nuts are high in fat (approximately 80 percent of their calories come from fat), but most of the fat is not saturated. Because nuts are high in calories, they should not be eaten in large amounts — generally no more than a handful a day.

Greek nuts are nutrient-dense foods rich in unsaturated fatty acids, protein, fiber, healthy minerals, tocopherols, phytosterols, and polyphenols.

TIP: Nuts found in Greece and the wider region include almonds, hazelnuts, pine nuts, pistachios, walnuts, and roasted chickpeas.

And why do Greeks snack on nuts so much? Again, it has to do with nuts positively affecting health outcomes. Even in ancient times, walnuts were said to be a gift to

Greece from Persia by the kings. Can you imagine the weight that walnuts carried for them to be considered for a royal present?

It's no surprise though when studies have associated nut consumption with a reduced incidence of coronary heart disease (in both sexes) and diabetes (only in women).[16] Randomized clinical trials demonstrate that nut intake has a cholesterol-lowering effect regardless of the background diet, and there is emerging evidence of beneficial effects on insulin sensitivity, oxidative stress, inflammation, and vascular reactivity.

Additionally, they have antioxidant action that contain a higher number of antioxidants than other foods. They are also a good source of omega-3 fats, can improve blood circulation, and protect against cardiovascular diseases.

They are also rich in essential minerals, such as calcium, magnesium, phosphorous, and potassium, whilst also promoting physical and mental development.

Another benefit is that this extra good fat that you gain from nuts may help you lose weight, or at least avoid gaining it. Studies have shown that vegetable fat may help to reduce body weight when these foods are

---

[16] Machado de Souza, Ravila. *Nuts and Human Health Outcomes: A Systematic Review*. MDPI, 2017. https://www.mdpi.com/2072-6643/9/12/1311

consumed in a healthy nutrition plan such as a SLOW Life diet.

TIP: Avoid candied, or honey-roasted, and heavily salted nuts. Opt-in for raw or roasted nuts and keep them unsalted, or at the very least, no salt added.

TIP #2: Aim to get 50 grams per day. Just use a small handful for your portions.

CHALLENGE: Snack on nuts. To keep yourself from reaching for unhealthy snacks, keep almonds, cashews, pistachios and walnuts on hand. Choose natural peanut butter, rather than the kind with hydrogenated fat added. Try tahini (blended sesame seeds) as a dip or spread for bread. And most importantly, swap sugar and fat loaded biscuits, crisps, and chocolate bars for these healthy snacks.

6. Village Habit 6: Grass Eater

Before you go to your backyard and start eating grass, read on to get a better understanding.

It's all about cereals. To give a little historical background of what cereals are, the word cereal translates from the Greek word *dimitriaka* which is derived from Demeter, the name of a Greek goddess of harvest and agriculture.

Cereals are grasses whose fruit or grains are edible. Examples of cereals are rice, barley, wheat and whole wheat, whole grains, rusks, corn or maize, durum wheat, oats, rye, millet, and wild rice.

TIP: There is a list of so-called pseudo-cereals which are now included in the list of cereals because they are utilized primarily as a staple food like cereals, although they are not grasses like cereals. These include quinoa, buckwheat, and grain amaranth.

So why are they so important to the Village lifestyle and nutrition? Cereals, or whole grains, in their natural form are packed with energy and vital nutrients. They are a vital source of carbohydrates, proteins, fats, minerals, vitamins, and phytochemicals – almost all types of nutrients. A major portion of cereals is carbohydrate, which makes cereals an economic source of food energy. They provide around 70-80% of an average person's daily energy requirement.

Cereals also contain essential minerals including phosphorus, potassium, magnesium, and calcium.

All these vital nutrients have been found from various studies to help lower cholesterol levels, increase blood vessel elasticity, aid various cellular metabolic activities, prevent heart attacks and cancer. Additionally, whole cereal foods, which are slowly digested, have a low glycemic index and are high in soluble fiber which helps prevent non-insulin dependent diabetes.

An important point about weight loss is that cereals are naturally low in fat, and with a high fiber content, are less energy dense. Hence, consumption of cereals, mainly sprouted cereals, help in weight loss. With a low glycemic index, as mentioned above, they provide a feeling of fullness and prevent overeating.

TIP: By making at least half of your grain choices whole grain, you'll enjoy the health benefits of dietary fiber and a host of disease-fighting nutrients. Choose a variety of whole grains each day. Aim to get around 70-80 grams per meal.

TIP #2: A great substitute to eating any type of breads is wheat rusk. Rusk is a double-toasted bread – it is hard and dry. In Greece, these are readily available and they are increasingly gaining popularity in other countries as well. If you cannot find these, look for a substitute like wholegrain complets of some kind of dry bread.

CHALLENGE: If you like cooking fried foods, why not combine wheat cereal and breadcrumbs to make a crunchy and fiber-filled fish or chicken breading. Or for breakfast, if you can't live without pancakes, add bran cereal/whole wheat flour to those homemade cakes for a hearty, filling breakfast.

7. Village Habit 7: Fish & Poultry

Conveniently close to the Mediterranean Sea, it's no surprise that Greeks eat mostly locally sourced seafood. In a village, a fisherman taking his *kaiki* in the early morning, fully decked with fishing nets and the steady yet muffled and meager sound coming from his engine of utility, is never far away, and you can not only see seasonal fish but also the catches of the actual day.

Seafood, both fish and shellfish, are consumed one to two times per week. Researchers in 2017 found that about 19.6 kilograms of fish (about 700 ounces) per annum is the average consumed by the Greeks whenever they eat seafood.

Why should we follow the lead of the Greeks and incorporate fish in our diets? Because they know that it is a low-fat, high-protein powerhouse packed with omega-3 fatty acids. Fish offers a wide range of health benefits, from keeping your brain and heart functioning properly to helping ease symptoms of depression, and even keeping your skin and hair looking radiant. However, you also get vitamins and minerals from seafood, such as vitamins A and C, magnesium, phosphorus, and selenium, to name a few.

The reason why this is important for you, and to understand the reason for fish being included in the SLOW Life diet, is the effect it has not only on your health, but also for weight loss. Omega-3s, as it was mentioned above, are fatty acids. Fatty acids are made up of a chain of carbon atoms, and they are a foundation of your body's ability to make fuel for itself. They essentially convert raw fuel into a refined and high energy source for your body. However, the body doesn't make essential fatty acids. It has to get it via the foods you eat, and fish has loads of them. This, combined with the combinations of proteins, allows you to feel fullers longer but not heavy or sluggish.

All these vitamins and nutrients have also led scientists to discover that consuming fish gives great health benefits. Fish may increase grey matter in the brain and protect it from age-related deterioration and is linked to reduced risk of autoimmune diseases, including type 1 diabetes. Fish also may help prevent asthma in children. It can protect your vision in old age and may improve sleep quality. One of the bigger benefits that the Mediterranean people find in fish is that it is easy to prepare and is very delicious.

TIP: Although fish in not a necessity in the diet in the strictest sense, it is still part of the lifestyle. It is not recommended that you eat fish every day, but if you are a fish lover, then eat at the recommended doses above (approximately 4 ounces per day up to 3 times weekly). Also, it should be noted that the Mediterranean fishermen do not overfish nor do the people overeat their seafood. The local fishermen cannot afford to ravage the local ecosystem so they fish seasonally. Additionally, the fish that the people consume are relatively small, such as sardines, anchovies, cod, as they are relatively inexpensive, found in abundance, and not exposed to high levels of mercury.

TIP #2: If you are not a fish lover, find a chef or restaurant that will prepare you a mild fish properly. Perhaps all these years you have been consuming fish the wrong way! Always get seasonal fish and try to consume as grilled, steamed, or shallowly fried.

TIP #3: Choose wild-caught fish over farmed. Wild fish tends to have more omega-3s and is less likely to be contaminated with harmful pollutants. If you have no other choice but to eat farmed fish, the benefits still far outweigh the risks. All types of fish are good for you, but if you can, choose wild-caught and ones that are in the middle of the food chain.

Fish and seafood in general are in the second level of the Mediterranean diet pyramid and this implies that they should be eaten relatively often, at most three times a week. And one of the common threads with the people that eat fish in the diet on a regular basis is that grilled or steamed, fish contains a minimum amount of fats that make it an ideal option for overweight people. Moreover, a fillet of any fish, sautéed in olive oil can double the nutrients that will not only keep you full for hours but nourish your cardiovascular health via promoting good cholesterol levels.

TIP: The Greeks eat fish all year round but tend to prefer the seasonal ones as they are the most likely to be caught fresh from the Mediterranean Sea. Seafood that is common in the SLOW Life diet are abalone, cockles, flounder, mackerel, octopus, sardines, sea bass, anchovies, squid (kalamari), cod.

Meat, on the other hand, is a food group that is eaten less in the Mediterranean region. There is a whole section dedicated to this later on so we will not get into detail at this point. However, if the Greeks consume meat, then poultry would be the most commonly eaten type of meat in the Village lifestyle diet, after fish.

When talking about poultry, we tend to think mostly of chicken. Indeed, it comes as no surprise that it is the most common type of meat under the poultry heading and what the Mediterranean people eat as well. However, what is interesting about the diet is that it does not only focus on chicken, but rather on the full range of poultry. This includes turkeys, pigeons, and upland game birds (quail, pheasant, partridges).

Although poultry should not be eaten on a regular basis, it still has some useful health benefits when consumed. A common thread with all poultry meat is that it is lean and high in protein. It also contains B vitamins in it which are useful for preventing cataracts and skin disorders, boosting immunity, eliminating weakness, regulating digestion, and improving the nervous system. Additionally, Vitamin D in poultry helps in calcium absorption and bone strengthening. Vitamin A helps in building eyesight and minerals such as iron are helpful in hemoglobin formation, muscle activity, and eliminating anemia. Potassium and sodium are electrolytes; phosphorus is helpful in tackling weakness, bone health, brain function, dental care, and metabolic issues.

Although not a main topic, eggs should be mentioned as well as they are a subsection of poultry.

Greeks usually eat eggs about three to four times per week. Specifically, they tend to usually fry an egg as a side dish with bread, sometimes almonds, and/or olives for breakfast, but also, they could eat as an omelet with vegetables. The eggs usually come from chickens that range freely, eat a wide variety of natural foods, and don't receive hormones or antibiotics. Slowly matured eggs are naturally higher in omega-3 fatty acids. Although not a staple to have at every meal in the SLOW Life diet, you can eat about three eggs per week.

8. Village Habit 8: No meat. No meat. What do you mean, he eat no meat?

Although it could be devastating to a Greek family when you tell them that you are vegetarian (just like in the film "My Big Fat Greek Wedding"), in the village, usually the lifestyle is that you are typically eating less red meat already. Historically, this was partly because it was harder and more expensive to graze and upkeep livestock, but also because fish and smaller animals, like poultry mentioned at number 6, were more abundantly available. Thus, eating meat tended to be saved for a celebratory meal.

The rule of thumb is to eat red meat only about once a week, but you can even make the rule for you to eat it every other week! Nevertheless, when the Greeks go and choose meats, they usually look for leaner cuts that will have less saturated fats. So, it would be good to brush up your knowledge on the anatomy of a cow to learn which are the leaner cuts.

More and more studies are showing that the consumption of meat, and more specifically red meat and processed meat, is associated with several chronic diseases. A new review of studies from Mayo Clinic showed that consumption of red meat and processed meat was associated with higher all-cause mortality, in other words higher risk of dying from all causes.[17]

TIP: Eating less meat, including processed meats, has two benefits: a reduced risk for certain forms of cancer, *and* a reduced effect on climate change. A report from the Intergovernmental Panel on Climate Change says switching to plant-based diets could both free up land and reduce carbon dioxide emissions.[18] Specifically, it calls for consumers to switch to diets featuring wholegrains, legumes and pulses such as lentils and chickpeas, fruit and vegetables. There are certain types of diets that have a lower carbon footprint and put less pressure on land. Dietary choices are very often shaped or influenced by local production practices and factors and cultural habits.

More specifically, most of the benefits that derive from the SLOW Life diet and lifestyle is evident from the reasons as to why you should *not* consume meat so often. A compound found in meat called carnitine has been found to cause atherosclerosis, the hardening or clogging of the arteries, according to a study in *Harvard*

---

[17] "Eating processed, red meats – what are the health risks?", https://newsnetwork.mayoclinic.org/discussion/mayo-clinic-q-and-a-eating-processed-red-meats-what-are-the-health-risks/
[18] https://www.ipcc.ch/srccl-report-download-page/

Health.[19] The research suggests that carnitine converts to a heart-damaging compound via bacteria in the intestine.

Another study found an association with red meat consumption and increased risk of a shortened lifespan. The cause is not clear, but it may be in the preparation, since charring meat increases toxins that can lead to cancer of the stomach.[20]

Also, meat contains a whole lot of iron which, when eaten in excess, can raise levels of iron in the brain and may increase the risk of developing Alzheimer's disease. When iron accumulates in the brain, a fatty tissue that coats nerve fiber is destroyed. This disrupts brain communication, and signs of Alzheimer's appear. As we already know from the above literature, the Village nutritional plan has shown that those who follow it have lower risk of developing Alzheimer's.

CHALLENGE: Although for some it may be difficult to go cold turkey (no pun intended) and decrease meat consumption to one day a week, start out by including meat as a side portion. So rather than eating a 5-6 ounce serving, cut down to 2 ounces of meat (approximately the size of a deck of cards or a bar of

---

[19] https://www.health.harvard.edu/healthbeat/whats-the-beef-with-red-meat
[20] *Dietary proteins and protein sources and risk of death,* The American Journal of Clinical Nutrition, V. 109, Issue 5, 2019.

soap) and fill the rest of the plate with vegetables and grains.

CHALLENGE #2: When making a sandwich, instead of using ham and cheese, you can make a cheese sandwich with the addition of plenty of vegetables, as well as healthy fats such as avocado or olive oil. You can even grill your vegetables, like sliced zucchini or eggplant, and have that in your sandwich with some sliced cheese. You can also use tahini or other nut butters in your sandwich to add a hint of protein and fat to your sandwich.

9. Village Habit 9: Liquid Therapy

Drink wine and live long! Yes, you read that right. Wine is part of the SLOW Life diet. If you look at the Mediterranean Diet Pyramid and related articles, it is mentioned that red wine can be taken in moderation daily. In the Greek culinary cuisine, wine accompanies any meal and many Greek recipes have wine, red or white, as one of the ingredients either as a marination or in cooking to release flavors in the dish.

When the SLOW Life diet refers to a glass of wine, it means red wine. Both red and white wines have phytonutrients, but white lacks some of the vital phytonutrients due to the process that is to make it. Red wine is made using the whole grape thus all phytonutrients of the grape are in the red wine.

The reason why Greeks drink red wine is because they know that wine fights diseases – in essence, it is a "healthy" alcohol! Studies have shown that wine contains flavonoids and non-flavonoids which in their turn contain antioxidants, and the antioxidants are the substances that have these healthy effects.[21]

Antioxidants are a variety of other substances like vitamins, phytonutrients, and minerals that prevent oxidation and specifically prevent the oxidation of cells and tissues. This has as the effect of preventing the

---

[21] "Wine Flavonoids in Health and Disease Prevention", https://www.ncbi.nlm.nih.gov/pmc/articles/PMC6155685/

destruction of the cells. This in turn prevents the blood from becoming sticky and thick which, as part of the chain effect, does not allow blood to clot thus reducing the risk of heart attack and stroke. [22] Antioxidants also boost the HDL cholesterol, known as ''good'' cholesterol and reduces the LDL cholesterol, known as ''bad'' cholesterol.

Wine, and more specifically red wine, prevents heart attacks because of the increased concentration of antioxidants it contains. Additionally, the antioxidants keep the immune system healthy, which in turn, acts as an anti-aging factor and fights infections and diseases.

TIP: As with every basic component in life, wine should be consumed in moderation since, apart from the antioxidants, wine is a source of calories. This is no difference for the SLOW Life diet. Thus, you should aim to consume approximately five ounces of dry red wine which only contains about 100 calories – the standard pour of a glass of wine.

TIP #2: Remember, the important point is that research on the Mediterranean diet shows that alcohol is generally consumed **with meals.** This is why Greeks see the full benefits of drinking wine and do not experience the adverse effects that it can have on the body if drunk in excess.

---

[22] Ibid.

CHALLENGE: If it's OK with your doctor, have a glass of wine at dinner. If you do not drink alcohol, you do not need to start. Instead, substitute it with purple/red grape juice, which is a good enough alternative to wine. Of course, if you are to drink a juice as a substitute, be sure to buy a natural, no added sugar juice.

10. Village Habit 10: Dairy and Greek Yogurt

Another main reason why the SLOW Life diet is one of the healthiest to follow is that dairy products have been part of it since the Neolithic period. The ancient Greeks even extolled the consumption of cheeses, and Hippocrates, in his treatises, described its medicinal benefits. However, the key when it comes to the diet is that there is not a major focus on them.

A recent study showed that the more servings of dairy foods adults consumed, the greater the percentage of their total calories that come from saturated fat (which is not a good thing). Therefore, when you do consume dairy products, you should choose low-fat dairy. Even though the low-fat option is not part of the SLOW Life diet in the traditional sense, I suggest it solely for caloric purposes while you can still maintain the health benefits, as it is readily available in supermarkets. Therefore, as you decrease the fat in dairy products, you cut calories, saturated fat, and cholesterol, while protein, calcium, and most other vitamins and minerals remain high, thus, still gaining the health benefits.

Health-wise, dairy products are one of the main food groups because they provide us, in addition to proteins and vitamins, the essential calcium that our body needs to replenish its bone system at any stage of human life. A diet rich in milk and dairy products is linked to increased bone health and a reduced risk of osteoporosis. Adequate milk intake is especially essential during childhood, as bone mass is still being built. Dairy is also associated with a reduced risk of type 2 diabetes, lowered blood pressure, and a decreased risk of cardiovascular disease in adults.

Because the SLOW Life diet is lower in dairy to begin with, and emphasizes consuming nuts as stated in habit number 5, individuals on a dairy-free diet can easily use dairy alternatives in their meals.

TIP: Milk spoils easily in the hot Greek climate, so the best way to preserve it is by turning it into cheese and yogurt. Cheese and yogurt were, and still are, traditionally eaten as an accompaniment to meals, which meant it was generally consumed in small amounts. Fortunately, Greek cheeses such as *kefalotyri* and *feta* are very rich in flavor, so a little goes a long way!

Greek yogurt is a main part of dairy consumption in Greece. A bowl of Greek yogurt can keep you fortified with essential nutrients and even help you lose weight.

Greek yogurt is a superfood partly due to the way it's made. It is made by straining out the extra whey in regular yogurt. It makes a yogurt that's thicker, creamier and tangier than regular yogurt. Plain Greek yogurt has less sugar and more protein than regular yogurt. But regular yogurt delivers twice the bone-strengthening mineral calcium. Greek yogurt also tends to be more expensive than regular yogurt, because more milk goes into making each cup.

Not only does Greek yogurt provide a healthy choice to include dairy in your diet, but it is also extremely healthy and is packed with probiotics.

Probiotics in the diet can enhance the good bacteria in the gut, improve health, and reduce the risk of certain diseases. They are great for the digestive system, and especially helpful to people who suffer from conditions such as irritable bowel syndrome. Without a healthy balance of good bacteria from probiotics, too much bad bacteria can build up and cause damage to our immune systems.

Apart from it being rich in probiotics, it is full of Vitamin B12, potassium (low in sodium), iodine which is important for a proper thyroid function – essential for a healthy metabolism, calcium, and packed with amino acids. All these have their own benefits that play a part in helping your body become healthier, but what they all do in tandem is that they play a major role in aiding you in losing weight.

TIP: Because Greek yogurt is thicker than regular yogurt, why not try to incorporate it into a smoothie drink? Alternately, you can use it as a topping on other foods. Use it as a substitute for sour cream, for dips, or as a sauce. You could also make your own frozen yogurt popsicles at home by freezing Greek yogurt mixed with fresh fruit.

CHALLENGE: Consume dairy in moderation. Limit higher fat dairy products such as whole or 2 percent milk, cheese, and ice cream. Switch to skim milk, fat-free yogurt, and low-fat cheese. Next time you have a craving for an ice-cream or for dips and sauces, reach for pudding made with skim milk and yogurt, respectively! They will go a long way in reaching your goal, in changing your lifestyle, and becoming healthier.

11. Village Habit 11: Spice Up Your Life

Although some romantic escapades would do you good in more ways than one, we are focusing on your eating habits!

This category I left for last because it's the part of adding flavor and panache to each one of your dishes. However, it is something not to be overlooked nor dismissed as unimportant. Herbs and spices growing in Greece are used in the culinary SLOW Life diet recipes not only to add taste but for health reasons as well.

Herbs and spices are an excellent substitute for blood pressure-raising sodium, with the added benefit of adding flavor and aroma to dishes. What's more, herbs and spices are chock full of antioxidants – key players when it comes to improving your heart health.

Herbs, and their derivatives, together with spices from trees and bushes, were collected and used when in season or they were dried to be used as and when needed.

TIP: The most abundant of the herbs and spices found in the Greek region and beyond are anise, basil, bay, capers, cardamom, cinnamon, chilis, chives, clove, coriander, dill, fennel, fenugreek, garlic, lavender, marjoram, mint, nutmeg, oregano, parsley, pepper, rosemary, saffron, sage, savory, sumac, turmeric, tarragon and thyme.

Although many believe that these do not add value to the dish. However, these simple seasonings actually spruce up the taste of dishes, and they contain phytochemicals, which are natural health-promoting substances that have been found to protect against conditions such as cancer and heart disease.

TIP #2: Introducing herbs and spices in dishes limits the salt you add on, which lowers sodium level intake.

A recent study in the USA revealed that out of top 50 antioxidant foods, five are spices and the leading antioxidant spice is oregano, a spice that originates from the Mediterranean basin. It was found that oregano has 4 times more antioxidant activity and benefits than blueberries!

The herbs and spices found in the SLOW Life diet have been shown in various studies to help with inflammation, to lower blood pressure, play a role in preventing the growth of cancer cells, fight off bacteria, and even protect against conditions that affect your brain or nervous system. Cinnamon has also been shown to lower blood sugar because it slows digestion, and therefore, the rise of blood sugar, which helps those people who have diabetes. One study that used turmeric revealed that even eating small amounts regularly may help prevent or slow down Alzheimer's disease, but also protect against arthritis, heart disease, and certain cancers.

Additionally, parsley is a rich source of the antioxidant Vitamin A and Vitamin C, providing protection from heart disease and cancer (and you thought eating your parsley garnish was a culinary sin!). Likewise, oregano is a nutrient-dense spice containing fiber, iron, manganese, calcium, Vitamin C, Vitamin A, and omega-3 fatty acids. It is also shown to have antibacterial and antioxidant properties. Even basil is known to have anti-inflammatory effects and may be useful for people with chronic inflammation, such as arthritis or inflammatory bowel disease. Basil also protects against bacteria and is an excellent source of Vitamin A, which helps reduce damage to the body from free radicals.

On the other hand, for weight loss, there is evidence that most of the herbs and spices have an effect in aiding you to shed off those excess pounds in various ways. Some boost your metabolism and help keep blood vessels healthy, others are naturally rich in iron (a lack of energy or feeling weak may be that you have iron deficiency), while all of them are low-in or have no calories at all.

TIP: Unless your doctor recommends otherwise, it's best to eat the herb or spice in its natural form rather than taking it in pill/supplement form. The compounds from herbs and spices you are eating with other foods work together to provide the extraordinary health benefits. Some work in tandem with others, being absorbed faster or releasing the precise doses that your body needs.

Herbal Teas

Although not part of the heading, I think teas deserve a mention. As stated previously, the health benefits of Greek herbs have been recognized for millennia, and to this day they continue to form the basis of folk remedies throughout the Greek countryside and villages. Many of these remedies are made by brewing teas from these herbal plants. There are some specific herbal plants that are predominately used as a tea and not as an ingredient or garnishes for enhancing food dishes. These are the ones I will focus on.

One of the most commonly found one is Greek mountain tea (*tsai tou vounou*). Its official Greek name *sideritis* (ironwort) literally means 'he who is made of, or contains iron'. Shaped like a spear with multiple yellow flowers, it grows at higher altitudes and has a mild and sweet aroma. As a remedy, it is one of the most potent antioxidants having antimicrobial and antifungal properties as well. It also helps ease stress and may help prevent cognitive disorders such as Alzheimer's and dementia.

Sage (or *faskomilo*) is also used for its tonic and anti-microbial properties. The fresh herb is commonly used in many savory dishes. Tea can be made from dried leaves although when brewed alone its somewhat peppery aroma can be rather intense, developing a bitterness if left to steep too long. As a remedy, it is thought to stimulate brain function and boost memory. It is also used to treat gastric imbalances, which also aids digestion and helps metabolism.

Louisa (or Lemon Verbena) is a widely grown herb. It has a calming effect and it is thought to help with balancing hormones. It is said to help combat fever and infections and aid in relieving indigestion, gassiness, and cramping. Louisa is also considered a good slimming aid as it helps curb and regulate the appetite. Indeed, some modern studies have lauded it as a perfect workout aid as its particular antioxidants are thought to protect and repair muscles damaged during exercise.

Chamomile is another common tea to drink while in Greece. The Greeks usually sweeten it with some homemade village honey, but it is also one of those cure-alls that people reach for whenever they are feeling under the weather. Chamomile is a mild sedative, can settle an upset stomach, and can act as a sleep aid. It also wildly grown in Greece and seems to do well in the climate.

Dittany, or *diktamo*, can be used as a herbal tea and its benefits are many. It is used for general healing, digestive issues, it is antimicrobial, antiseptic, anthelmintic, anti-hemorrhagic, emmenagogue, antispasmodic, it soothes stomach aches and relieves nausea, and has antiepileptic properties. Dittany has been the subject of study and much modern scientific research. The main components of its essential oil (contains over 40 different ingredients with predominantly carvacrol and cumin) but also the number of flavonoids that have been isolated and identified are responsible for the medicinal properties of the plant. Its aroma is very intense, so many villagers add in honey to sweeten it up.

CHALLENGE: Most Americans consume about 1,000 mg of sodium over the amount recommended by nutrition and health experts. New research shows cooking with spices and herbs could help you ditch the salt shaker and meet sodium recommendations. When it comes to heavy creams and sauces, swap them with herbs and spices.

CHALLENGE 2: Add oregano, crushed garlic and red pepper to no-salt added tomato sauce for a tasty, low-sodium pasta dinner.

CHALLENGE 3: Look to add variety to your beverages by drinking hot or cold tea with herbs.

12. Village Habit 12: Your Body is a Wonderland

This section has three subheadings to it. They are each nonetheless very important to help with you losing weight and getting you on the path to a healthier lifestyle. They all have to do with looking after your body which is the ultimate instrument that needs to looked after as well.

The habits described below are already part of the Village lifestyle, so they will aid you in your journey to fully integrate the habits in your life and routine. And no, none of them have anything to do with John Mayer serenading to you.

A. Binge Drinking

The first part of the extra habits to incorporate is to drink lots and lots of water (What, you thought that the title meant something else?). But what in essence does drinking lots of water mean? Although everyone has different needs, nutritionists say that sticking to the oft-recommended amount of eight 8-ounce glasses (64 ounces total) should suffice and can help boost weight loss for the average person or someone just looking to drop a few pounds. I was told by my nutritionist to drink 3 liters (about 101 ounces total) per day. So, I would say to use the two numbers as a minimum-maximum range.

However, the problem is not actually drinking this amount, as it doesn't sound like an overwhelming number, but the challenge for most people is drinking enough water in the first place.

TIP: If you're a gym rat or endurance athlete, you'll need more water than the standard 64 ounces. Be sure to get the required amount that your body needs.

Right about now, although you may have heard of the notion that drinking water will help you lost weight, you are probably wondering why this is the case. The simple answer is that water helps the metabolic process. You brain does not distinguish between food and water and treats water as food. This means that the metabolic process is kick started as soon as you drink water and will start to use the energy to process the water.

To give you a simple explanation, the metabolism of fat – the one we are interested in losing – is processed by the liver when it converts stored fat to energy. If you are not drinking enough water, the kidneys are not functioning properly, and the liver must pick up the slack of the improperly functioning kidneys, which in turn lowers the proper operation of the liver. Thus, the liver cannot metabolize fat as quickly as it should and fat is stored.

TIP: If you're feeling quenched, be sure not to overdo it; drinking too much water could lead to hyponatremia, also known as water intoxication.

TIP #2: When you crave eating or drinking, or just doing merely out of habit, a sugary and caloric beverage, choose water instead – it will save you a lot of unnecessary calories. Soft drinks, which account for about half of an average consumer's sugar intake, are a main reason for people having an unhealthy lifestyle. Greeks do not drink many soft drinks, instead they opt for water, coffee, tea, and red wine.

A few other benefits of drinking plenty of water are that it will flush out impurities and will leave your skin glowing and looking younger and healthier; it will aid your muscle tone by allowing you to work our more effectively as muscles will contract easier. It is also said that water facilitates blood flow and lessens the chance of a blood clot.

B. Sweet Dreams

The second part of the extra benefits is to tuck in and go to dreamland more often. Train your body to sleep more during the night and to take a nap during the day.

But how does sleeping and taking naps relate to losing weight and having a healthy lifestyle? Research shows that the rise in obesity over recent decades has been accompanied by a growth in chronic sleep problems. The Greeks found out long ago that napping was a medicine on its own. It was not a sign of laziness or lethargy. Sleep actually plays a key role in maintaining health, including managing our weight, and lack of sleep is a known risk factor for obesity.

A Harvard Public School study revealed that Greeks, in the control group, who took regular 30-minute naps or siestas were 37 percent less likely to die of heart disease over a six-year period than those who never napped.[23] That's a staggering amount! Sleep at any time of the day acts like a valve to release the stress of everyday life. That's what happens at night and why our body needs the rest. It restores itself after a long day of external bombardment on our system. Imagine then what a nap could do during the day. Blood pressure is reduced and heart rates slow. At the same time, the immune system restores itself. Increasingly, researchers are recognizing the role the immune system plays in heart disease, and without a healthy functioning immune system, your heart could be at risk.

Although it may be difficult to do this on a daily basis, especially if you are living an urban lifestyle, it is worth trying to incorporate it in some alone time, for example during the weekends. Instead of turning on the tv and

---

[23]

https://www.recoveryonpurpose.com/upload/Siestas%20and%20Your%20Heart.pdf

"vegging-out", try to put your feet up on the sofa or your bed, read a good book, and then let your eyes drift away into dreamland for a short period in the afternoon, which will split your day up to two. But do not turn a nap into a short sleep cycle as this will mess with your circadian sleep cycle and throw off your nightly schedule. If you do this, then you will feel well refreshed after waking up, with extra energy to tackle the rest of the day!

Generally, less sleep allows your hunger hormones to kick into gear. To put it simply, shorter sleep duration has been found to lead to the body increasing its energy intake by eating more food. Even a single night of sleep deprivation can make you feel hungrier and more likely to make bad food choices, thus, increasing your desire for high-calorie, weight-gain promoting foods, i.e. junk food.

The other effect that sleep-deprivation has on a body is that it can cause your core body temperature to drop lower than it should. You see, over the course of a 24-hour period, our body temperature fluctuates in accordance with in-built circadian rhythms. This drop in body temperature could cause the body to use up energy stores to thermoregulate, leaving a person more tired and drained.

Lastly, chronic sleep deprivation causes daytime fatigue, which in turn promotes obesity by discouraging exercise and other calorie-burning activities. Couple this with the increase in consuming higher-caloric foods, and you have a recipe for gaining weight success.

TIP: Not only are workouts more likely to occur when you are rested but they also tend to be more vigorous with increased energy. Along with exercise burning off calories, gaining strength through resistance training can increase metabolism. And not to mention, staying active and partaking in workouts further heightens energy levels.

Following this, one of the most important sleep activities that Greeks do is siesta, i.e. taking a nap during the day.

After the explanation above, it is understandable that losing sleep at night affects how your metabolism functions. But, how does a nap help you through the day and to lose weight? Well, there has also been much research that breaking up your day with a nap has tremendous benefits to your health, your lifestyle, and your goal to lose weight.

Though the desire of a midafternoon snack may be related to hormones and the desire for a pick-me-up, taking a 20-minute nap can distract against those munchies. Nutrition experts truly encourage individuals to recognize whether or not they are experiencing true hunger or cravings, further recommending a plan of action to divert boredom-based eating. Relaxing and taking a nap is a valuable way to sidetrack from food.

Additionally, emotions can be heightened when tired, ultimately slowing down metabolism and dumping out harmful chemicals in times of stress. More specifically, increased release of cortisol can contribute to weight gain in the abdominal region and trigger cravings towards high-carbohydrate products, as such foods have shown to induce a calming effect. So, not only can taking a nap sidetrack from food but it can also combat emotions that may initiate a craving.

TIP: A study done with Greeks found that those who took a 30-minute nap at least three times a week had 37% less risk of dying from a heart-related condition. Among working men their risk of death was reduced 64%!

C. Fresh Air

Greeks spend a lot of time outdoors, whether they are running errands, doing work, eating, being active, or just spending time with friends and/or family. But how does this help you to slim down and lead a healthy lifestyle?

It is down to the simple fact that being in nature, being outdoors, is an uplifting experience on its own. Just being happy and content with the moment you are experiencing releases certain happy hormones, specifically serotonin. Your uplifting mood will change the way you act, react, think, and will give you positive energy to do more, thus, creating a chain reaction with your activity and lifestyle.

From a scientific viewpoint, researchers have found that daylight can kick-start a fat burning mechanism in the body. A particular type of fat known as brown adipose tissue (or BAT) transfers energy into heat and this boosts calorie burning. The scientists found that by spending time outside, mostly where it is cooler than room temperature, this energy-to-heat reaction is boosted and so dieters lose weight.[24]

TIP: Winter was traditionally a time of the year that was accompanied with increased thermal demands and thus energy expenditure, but the body's requirements for brown fat has been reduced in recent times by central heating and the effects of global warming. Along with the cooling of the air, as a reaction, our bodies feel the need to eat. Under this behavior, there is a need for energy. The energy need due to feeling cold is met with food. That is why usually in the winter

---

[24] University of Nottingham. "Daylight Could Help Control Our Weight." ScienceDaily. ScienceDaily, 25 August 2009. www.sciencedaily.com/releases/2009/08/090821135024.htm

time, we gain weight compared to the summer time (see below).

In the summertime, on the other hand, sunshine not only lifts the mood (see above), but researchers have found that it also shrinks fat cells. In the *Scientific Reports,* it was reported that when the sun's blue light wavelengths—the light we can see with our eye—penetrate our skin and reach the fat cells just beneath, lipid droplets reduce in size and are released out of the cell.[25] In other words, our cells don't store as much fat. As stated above, countless studies have shown the importance of water when it comes to weight loss, especially before every meal. In the summer, it necessitates drinking more water, leading to a feeling of satiety and consuming less food.

However, summer can also be a psychological motivating factor as it means short skirts, sleeveless tops, and swimming costumes. We all want to be in great shape and feel confident. However, some women consider wearing a bikini a bigger threat to their confidence than baring all in the bedroom. Thus, the desire to wear revealing outfits that allow us to feel confident and happy in our skin is a serious motivation to make these changes in our lives.

The bottom line is to spend as much as time outdoors as you possibly can! It will not only boost your energy,

---

[25] Sandoiu, Ana, "Weight loss breakthrough: Sunlight is key." Medical News Today, 11 January 2018. https://www.medicalnewstoday.com/articles/320592.php

mood and mind, but it will also help burn fat and shrink fat cells.

VI. Lifestyle change

Making a lifestyle change is challenging, especially when you want to transform many things at once. A key mental note is not to think of it as a resolution but rather as an evolution.

Lifestyle changes are a process that take time and require support. It happens on an incremental basis and not overnight. This is why it is an evolution: it is a process of gradual change over time. Once you are ready to make a change, then you make resolutions about the things you want to change, but the difficult part is actually committing and following through. Having looked at the SLOW Life diet and the habits that we have to implement, we should understand why a Greek village lifestyle change is so important.

The secret to improved health is to make subtle but permanent changes to your attitude towards food and exercise. There is no point in trying to dramatically change your nutritional habits and do lots of exercise if you are only going to keep it up for a few days or for a short period of time. You will find it easier to keep your new resolutions by making small changes that suit your lifestyle and naturally become part of your routine.

To desire a change in lifestyle for health reasons means that you want more out of life. By choosing to read this book, you have made a commitment to exploring the SLOW Life diet. You crave to be closer to nature, to be closer to family and friends, to eat healthy, and exercise by moving more. You will still not feel comfortable in your own skin if you cannot accept yourself the way you are. A change of appearance does not mean anything unless there is a change of the mind.

That's why when I started my journey to lose weight and lead a healthier life, my mindset had to change so I could successfully accomplish my goals. I had programmed myself to make the change because this "diet" is largely based on a certain lifestyle and implementing the habits that make this healthier lifestyle such a success. All this starts with the mind.

However, to make my decision was, on the one hand, an easy one, yet on the other, it was actually rather difficult. It was an easy decision because my cardiologist, who told me at my check-up that if I did not make a change in my life to lose weight, then he could not guarantee that in the next check-up, he would be able to give me good news. In other words, I was on the verge of something potentially irreversible and disastrous to myself and to the ones around me. It thus made it an easy decision for me because I have a family – a wife and two young children. It became an easy decision because I did not like the way I felt and looked.

On the other hand, it was a difficult decision because I was scared; scared of the unknown. It was a difficult decision because I doubted myself: did I have the inner strength to achieve the goal that was at the end of a, now, one-way street? It was a difficult decision because I felt powerless.

All these external factors, what I call the environmental factors, make your decision easy. On the other side of the coin, all the internal factors, what I call the emotional factors, make your decision the most difficult one you will make.

To make sense of my internal factors and to assess each one and its importance, I performed what I call a thought map. Although it is a mental exercise, it is helpful to put it on paper and to visualize these emotions and feelings. It will give you a better picture of what is going on inside you.

When I made the decision to change my lifestyle and become healthy, I sat down to make a mental assessment of my current lifestyle. I exercised my mental mind mapping skills and put it to use. This exercise allowed me to realize and conceptualize my habits.

TIP: Although I did this exercise mentally, if it helps you to write it down, do so. Here is what a mind map looks like. What I realized was that there were a couple of obvious changes I needed to make but some were not so obvious but became clear after I manifested my mind map into a visual aid.

MINDMAP

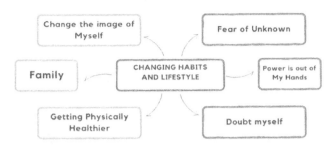

The mind map, or thought map, can be as comprehensive as you like or as limited as you like. The branching thoughts stemmed from the core thought because they related to each other. As a general rule, the ones stemming from the central box should be core, estuary thoughts and anything from that can branch out into related but separate thoughts. I also color coded the thoughts: blue for positive feeling, red for negative feeling. You can choose any colors you like. More times than not, if you have been held back from achieving your goals, your thought map will have more negative feelings than positive ones. By putting them on paper, you are able to tackle them one-by-one.

TIP: An effective way to promote behavioral change is to set goals and make plans. Once you described and identified, from your mind map, the thoughts on your current lifestyle, you should then make your goals be clear and specific, describing the what, where, and when of any given behavior. These goals are better when they are specific, measurable, attainable, relevant, and timely.

The one obvious change in my lifestyle that I had to implement immediately after looking at my mind map and assessing my situation at that time of my life, was to re-introduce activity back into my weekly routine. Although I had a busy schedule – working late hours and any free time I had wanting to spend it with my family – I had to find something that would fit into my program.

I highly recommend finding an exercise group and joining it. Ideally, this group will have like-minded people participating and trainers who understand your plight and situation and encourage you to reach your goals. But be cautious where you choose your group. Try to find one outside of a gym. This is because when you sign up for a group or with a trainer, you become financially committed, and thus, psychologically, this commitment will encourage you to go, as a high financial burden placed on every training session (as opposed to a gym with an annual membership fee where it is a miniscule financial burden apportioned to each session you go to over the course of a year) will give you an extra incentive to push and motivate yourself to go.

You can also share your goals as this would create a psychological contract with them, which makes the goals harder to break. Additionally, you eventually create a familial bond with this group, again, as opposed to a gym where you fall into the membership oblivion and never create a strong bond with staff and other gym goers. This goes to the notion that one of the main reasons why people do exercise is that it provides social contact which results in motivation.

Exercise is more likely to happen if it is a social activity which brings with it social benefits. Not recognizing or valuing the social benefits of exercise may lead to people becoming inactive, which in turn can prompt weight gain.

Regarding my personal experience, I have tried all sorts of gyms and training facilities. I almost gave up finding something that I not only liked and which motivated me to go, but also to create that bond with like-minded people. I eventually found a group that had a training program which seemed to have what I was looking for: the right program, the right messages that are delivered to the customers, and the right time slots that fit my schedule. However, I still had to try them out and see if we would truly be a fit.

I assessed their schedule and decided to go to my first session. It ended up being the 7:15 a.m. slot, and it fell on a windy autumn morning, still dark outside, and it turned out that although a daunting task to push yourself to get out of bed and venture out that early for something unknown, ended up being exactly what I was looking for.

This "gym" was outdoors. The program was a hybrid of cross-training and circuit training, and the trainers, and other participants, encouraged and pushed each other to get results. Thus, I committed myself, both mentally and physically, to two days a week of exercise as a start since I was making a change in my life, one that required dedication and commitment. Albeit a small commitment of only two days, that was what I could give at that time. But that's ok. Baby steps allowed me to not be overwhelmed and to adjust my life and schedule as I progressed through my journey. It also created a routine in my lifestyle which becomes hard to break further down the road.

TIP: When involving yourself in something new to determine whether it will become part of your routine, start off slow. Baby steps help you get used to the new idea and not to be overwhelmed, to make it part of your routine and to ease you into your new schedule. Once it is a part of your life and routine, then you can ramp up your efforts. In other words, a habit will be established which increasingly becomes difficult to break in the future.

At the new training facility and program, the trainers knew what I wanted to achieve after discussing with them my concerns, fears, and goals; moving forward, they continuously monitored the progress I was making as well as encouraged me to keep going. This helped my mental state and motivation because even as winter rolled in and I was waking up before sunrise, while the cold penetrated my bones, I was determined to get it done.

I found motivation in the little things that I was achieving: booking my morning sessions via the online app, waking up and getting dressed, opening the front door, or even just making the decision to go. I felt better every time I went, even though my muscles were aching in different parts of my body that I didn't even know I had, let alone use! However, slowly, I realized that I had more energy to tackle the tasks of the day; I was more efficient while maintaining a level of stamina that drove me forward. All the pain I endured in the beginning was telling me to quit and just stay in bed. But I persevered. And as time progressed, it became easier. More importantly, after the effort that I put in, a reaction occurred, my weight and fat started dropping, albeit slowly, but still surely.

TIP: Productivity makes you feel happy and gives you motivation. When you are productive in a something you enjoy doing, your brain releases dopamine which helps push that motivation. Procrastination, on the other hand, stems from being distracted from seemingly mundane and repeated tasks that do not challenge you. This in turn makes you feel worse inside as it triggers in your brain the feeling of guiltiness and shame. Once you have felt the psychological benefits of being productive, for example doing exercise, then you will start to believe that being active benefits you and therefore you will do more of it.

After several months of doing this routine, I had lost approximately 5 kilograms, but this was not enough for me. I had to step it up if were to achieve my goals. I set up a meeting with my trainers and told them what I really wanted to achieve. The trainers and I set up a program that seemed to have what I was looking for to accelerate my weight loss by shedding fat and putting on muscle while simultaneously alternating my eating lifestyle. We increased my training schedule to three days per week and began a nutrition program based on the SLOW Life diet and local foods.

I was focused and determined to achieve my goal. I then took the next step in my journey: I started my nutrition program. In so doing, I prepared my wife and family: for the next two months, I would be fully engaged with the program.

Advice Tip: As our behaviors are intricately linked with other people, if we try to change our behavior, these other people in our lives may object and the pressure is on to behave the way we have always done, sliding back into our old habits and lifestyle. Remember, people like us to carry on the way we always have done as it makes them feel safe. If we change, then they may feel they have to change, and that is unsettling.[26] Therefore, it is best to psychologically prepare anyone to the changes you will make around the house, including your meal plan– you do not want to surprise them with your new regime. Do not forget to also prepare yourself. It will be a significant change not only to you but also to the ones around you.

As you may have guessed, after three weeks, my wife wanted me to stop and reassess my eating plan. She saw this as a burden, not on me, but on her and the children. She expressed this by saying that I needed to eat different type of foods and vary my nutrition. She felt that my nutrition regime was monotonous, and it became a problem to cook different meals all the time!

However, I let her know I was determined to continue. Instead of just asking my wife to bear my lifestyle

---

[26] Ogden, Jane. *The Psychology of Dieting.* Routledge, London, p. 46.

regime, I asked her to join in and be a part of the habit changes I was making. Either way, almost a month had gone by and I was going to stick with it. Of course, any support and encouragement to keep me going until the end of the two-month period would go a long way towards helping me reach my goal. I wanted to reach the finish line, and I was going to do it. She understood how determined I was and the importance of having a support network throughout this journey. In the end, not only did she support me, she also adopted many of the eating habits as well.

TIP: When changing our eating habits, we also have to be able to manage our home environment. It involves self-monitoring, goals and routine to manage it successfully when in this transition phase. First, only food that you plan to eat should be brought into the house. If you don't want to eat it, don't buy it. Thus, plan your meals for the week, write a list, and buy the ingredients and bring them home. Second, choose a place to eat in your home – do not choose this place to be in front of the computer or TV. Wherever you choose, this should be the go-to place associated with eating.

Lastly, choose when to eat. Ideally, it should be three proper meals and perhaps two in between snacks. Eat dinner early rather than late and make that your final meal of the day. Soon, it will become a habit through repetition and not only will your stomach get used to it, but you will also feel like it is a part of your new lifestyle.

Fast forward to about a month later, I completed the program and went to my nutritionist to record my progress measurements. To my surprise, although I felt better and could feel that a change had occurred, it is different to see it as something tangible. The results were better than expected – I had lost 8 kg, reduced my body fat by 5% and had dropped 2 inches off my waist line. And although it is not an east task to continue doing this as the temptations are always there to bring you down, it gets easier as the routine becomes a part of your lifestyle.

TIP: It's important to find a training group that you identify with. I found a training group which suited not only my personality but also reflected where my life was at the time and what I wanted to achieve (see Tip #2 below) It was also in close proximity to my house which allowed me to not use my car. I was able to walk there and get in a little exercise (and to clear my mind) even before my training!

TIP #2: Let your trainer and workout group know why you decided to come and join and what you want to achieve. They will then give you the support and motivation you need when things get tough and you feel you want to give up. Believe me, in the beginning, you will have days where you will want to pack your bags and quit. However, the trainers should not only understand your strife, embrace your goals, and keep you motivated at every step of the way, but also the rest of the participants should also reflect the ethos of the place and be encouraging because they are going through the same struggle as you, each on a different level of course, but still fighting their own battles. And the best part about the training group I found: we did our exercise outdoors, come rain or shine!

TIP #3: It is easier to make these changes with your partner or a friend, especially if they live in the same household as you. That way, you can encourage each other as well as have that mental support that is much needed when going through a lifestyle change.

VII. Bonus Material: Making Lifestyle Changes that Lead to Lasting Habits

Make a plan. Your plan is a map that will guide you on this journey of change. When making your plan, be specific. Want to exercise more? Detail the time of day when you can take walks and how long you'll walk. Write everything down, and ask yourself if you're confident that these activities and goals are realistic for you. The idea is to fulfil each step on your plan to achieve maximum change.

Baby Steps. After you've identified realistic short-term and long-term goals, break down your goals into small, manageable steps that are specifically defined and can be measured. Don't bite a bigger piece than you can handle because that will set you up for failure.

Change one habit at a time. Unhealthy behaviors develop over the course of time, so replacing unhealthy habits with healthy ones requires time. Many people run into problems when they try to change too much too fast. To improve your success, focus on one goal or change at a time. As new, healthy behaviors become a habit, try to add another goal that works toward the overall change you're striving for.

Involve your loved ones. Whether it be a friend, co-worker or family member, someone else on your journey will keep you motivated and accountable. Having someone with whom to share your struggles and successes makes the work easier and the mission less intimidating. Not only involve them, but also share with them your experiences. If you have children, make it a game with the whole family and tell them they can be your coaches in creating these habits, eating right, and being healthier. Once they are involved, they will pick up the habits and acquire new tastes in their eating habits. I found that when I involved my whole family, not only my success rate increased, but also my wife's did as well and my children became happier to be involved.

Habits are formed through four processes: modelling, repetition, reinforcement, and association. When we repeat a behavior several times, it becomes a pattern. It then becomes a habit if it is reinforced by something positive such as the fact that we like it, that someone else likes us doing it and that makes you feel good.[27]

The Last Mile

Why is the Greek Village lifestyle something you should incorporate into your life? Greeks live this life because they were born into it, they grew up with it, it is part of being. However, for you, it is important, because this lifestyle has been proven to be healthy and life-altering by researchers and scientists alike. The diet has produced astonishing results in scientific studies showcasing a number of health benefits. This way of

---

[27] Ibid, p. 42.

life has been associated with longevity and overall health happiness.

Why was it important for me to tell you my story? Why was it important for me to share with you my grandmother's life routine? Because it showcased and highlighted the steps that you must go through to implement changes in your life to achieve your goals. To make the lifestyle change that the SLOW Life diet requires, it is imperative to have a clear path and plan in mind and then to take baby steps to give yourself the tools to succeed, one step at a time. The success is not determined by one incident, but it is achieved from all the previous steps you take, culminating in that last breakthrough.

One of my favorite stories about the stonecutter, shows you exactly what I describe above:

"When nothing seems to help, I go back and look at the stonecutter hammering away at his rock perhaps a hundred times without as much as a crack showing in it. Yet at the hundred and first blow, it will split in two, and I know it was not that blow that did it – but all that had gone before."

This quote was made by Jacob Riis, an immigrant from Denmark who arrived in New York City as a 21-year-old in 1870 with $40 in his pocket. He became a police photographer and became friends with the NYC Police Commissioner and future President Theodore Roosevelt. After seeing major poverty in the neighborhoods, Riis became a social reformer who published a photography book called "How the other half lives." This book was so influential that "it inspired Roosevelt to close the worst of the lodging houses and spurred city officials to reform and enforce the city's housing policies."[28]

This quote embodies the very essence of anyone's effort in any endeavor undertaken. It can be learning a musical instrument, learning mathematics, cooking, going to medical or engineering school, or even just figuring out how to work the dishwasher in your house. If you cannot solve or figure it out, you do not give up, but you just keep looking, keep trying, and keep going. Eventually, that last blow will break the stone.

This concept is important to understand because in order for my story and this book to resonate and be useful for you, you will have to start with the notion that *you* will have to change. You must not only make the decision to want to go down this path and to start incrementally implementing these changes, pounding the rock one blow at a time, but also your whole mindset will need to follow suit to buy-in for what you want to achieve.

For your mindset to follow suit and change, it is imperative that you strip-down all the preconceptions of who you think you are. The critical thing that you need to get going is to surrender all your limitations. The idea

---

[28] Leadership Case Studies: The Leadership Lessons of Gregg Popovich. 2015.

is to give up on all the notions that you have placed on yourself about what you are capable of.

What this means is that when you search and delve into your past, all these ideas and notions you have labeled yourself with must be discarded. For example, perhaps in your past you have said to yourself, "I can't possibly learn that", or "I'm not adventurous", or "I can't play any instrument", or "I can't draw", or "I can't possibly lose weight", or whatever else the case may be, are all the limitations which result in restricting you from achieving what you want. And these were probably fixed on you somewhere in the past by someone or even yourself.

These limitations are as real as you make them – they become the reality that you mold them to be. Any bad things that have happened in your life, you picked up this idea that these bad things define you, and thus, are a part of you. This includes bad habits like binge eating or drinking. Regardless of whether you wanted to or not, you pick up these ideas and they become intertwined with you as a learner. That is why it is important for you to drop these limitations that you *believe* define you.

Behavior and lifestyle are directly linked to your general wellbeing and body weight. Once you start believing this, and not that it is the fault of some external factor, you will feel less powerless and hopeless over your weight and more likely to succeed in making a true difference in and to your life.[29] Believing that things can change is a powerful tool to give you the motivation that you seek.

You will start to think differently and start to take on positive ideas about yourself because you *are* able to make these lifestyle changes, you *are* able to adopt these habits, you *are* disciplined enough to lose weight, and you *are* capable of being happier and healthier. This is *you*.

What's stopping you in making these changes in your life? The simple answer is excuses. I've heard - and have used myself – the following excuses one too many times: "Oh, I don't have time", or "Oh, I don't have enough money", or "Oh, I don't have the right resources". Given that we live very much in the moment, at the time of choosing to be active or when applying a habit in your life, the benefits at that precise moment need to outweigh the costs.[30] This is when a mental bond will form between that activity or habit and positivity. However, what happens is that many costs get in the way and this is exactly when people start using excuses. It's easier to make an excuse to give yourself an 'out' than to work out a way to find a solution to meet that challenge head-on; in essence though, the only thing that stops you is *you*. It's the mindset of a procrastinator.

_____

[29] Ogden, Jane. *Ibid,* p. 78.
[30] Ogden, Jane. *Ibid,* p. 26.

If you sit down and ponder about any excuses you have used recently, you will see that all excuses are fabricated. They are, in essence, lies that you create to convince yourself that you cannot or will not do whatever it is you would like to do, something in which you can find your greatness. To fight these lies though, you need the truth. But what could possibly be the truth? Whatever problem you have in your life, whatever excuse you use which holds you back from achieving your goals, for you to be reading this book means that there is something you do want to change in your life.

At the end of the day, no one truly wants to hear your sob stories because everyone has their own problems to deal with as well. Thus, stop the pouting and get to work to change your life. Part of losing weight and restructuring your lifestyle for the longer term is the establishment of a new healthier routine which can persist forever onwards rather than just in the shorter term. You have to change the way you are eating and live for a life; it is not for a period but it is permanent.

In your journey of this lifestyle change, make every day count because there is only one of you, there is only one life to live, and there is only one now. Every day that passes is gone. Make your goal a part of you and be relentless in achieving that dream. There will be distractions, like TV, your phone, your friend(s), and/or your family, but do not waste time in succumbing to these, instead, persevere for what you want to achieve.

You only have one life to accomplish what you want, and the only time to fulfill your goals is now.

Conclusion

Congratulations for taking new steps to changing your life.

Each day is but a series of conflict between the right way and the easy way. And your choice to make the change is a path headed upstream. Leading the same lifestyle that has gotten you here is comfortable and safe. To turn your back on these is the choice you make, but that's only the first step – from here, it only gets tougher because your fears, doubts, and insecurities are always going to be there to turn you around to the path of your old lifestyle, the one that is comfortable. But you can defeat them by listening to your body, your mind, and your heart.

About the Author

I was born and raised in Natchez, Mississippi. My parents originated from the island of Lesvos, Greece, and we moved back to Greece when I was twelve years old.

I am a lawyer and social entrepreneur who started my business path with reviving my family tradition of olive oil production on the island of Lesvos, Greece, with my company evo3 olive farms. Through my love and knowledge of olive oil, I began to advocate for its health benefits and the role it played in the Mediterranean diet. I not only promoted olive oil's health benefits, but also saw that the Greek village diet was much more than just food, but a lifestyle, and I witnessed first-hand that it could make someone live longer, happier, and healthier.

I am the founder and CEO of evo3 olive farms. This company was the first Greek social enterprise in the olive oil sector which paved the way for other producers to look at the circle economy as a viable solution. I work with Eden Reforestation Projects with the tree planting in Africa and Haiti. For every bottle sold, we plant a tree in a deforested area. By teaming up with Eden, evo3 olive farms not only plants trees - through its valued customers and partner - but also gives work to impoverished local people dedicated to earn a supplemental income by planting these trees and reviving their local forests and farmlands. My company exports the olive oil, which can be found mostly in the United States, the United Kingdom, and in the BeNeLux region.

The olive oil we produce is a 3rd generational family tradition which stemmed back to my grandfather. It has a deep meaning to me and how I carry the tradition forward to continue the legacy. My grandfather, Ioannis Kamatsos, farmer and father of five, bore the winters and fought off starvation during World War II to produce olive oil, his most precious commodity. He would load his oil onto a small fishing boat in the middle of the night, crossing the Aegean Sea to the mainland, evading German and Italian soldiers, risking his life for his family, to trade his valuable olive oil for enough food and supplies to keep them alive during the harsh times of the war.

My father, George, immigrated to the United States by himself when he became of legal age, trading his father's olive trees for knowledge in medicine. After 27 years in the United States, his return to his native island brought an intense desire to pick up where his father had left off. Transforming the production to organic cultivation using sustainable methods, he also continued to use the traditional methods that he had learned from his father. I then took the reins from my father.

Our family's olive oil has won many taste and branding awards, including from the New York International Olive Oil Competition, the Los Angeles International Olive Oil Competition, the London Great Taste awards, and the AVPA olive oil competition in France. I am an olive oil sommelier, giving olive oil taste lectures on how to taste olive oil and choosing the right one, and also the benefits of using olive oil and the role it plays in the Mediterranean diet.

I was also a TedX speaker. My talk focused on creating a business based on social value rather than only financial value. It is called, "Entrepreneurship and Empathy". Please turn on the subtitles as the original language is Greek.

I have recently co-founded another business, Ethically Sourced For You, focusing on ethical and sustainable goods and products and changing the way we shop and how retailers buy their products.

I have been an advocate for the Greek and Mediterranean lifestyle and diet which has transformed my life. It was a transformation not only of the body, but of the mind, soul, and his values. I wanted to share this journey with you.

Final words

I want to thank you again for downloading this book and taking the first steps toward your goals and changing your lifestyle!

I really hope that I was able to help you understand the best way to implement the SLOW Life diet lifestyle, provide helpful tips in doing this, and solutions to achieve what you personally set out.

What you should do now is test the habits and implementation tips in this book and let me know how effective they are in overcoming current unhealthy lifestyle and habits.

And if you get a chance to visit Greece, go to a village, stay there, take in the scenery, enjoy the smells, the tastes, the sounds, meet the people, live their way of life, and most importantly, learn from them. Remember, you have one life, fully embrace that you hold your destiny in your hands; make it count.

REVIEW

Did this book help you in some way? Did you learn something? If so, I would love to hear about it. Honest reviews help readers find the right book for their needs and I enjoy reading them as I can learn from them as well. You can post a review on the Amazon book page.

Thank you.

COMPLIMENTARY MENU FOR FREE

As a sign of my appreciation, and to get you started on your journey, I put together a 1-week menu that is nutritional as well as based on the Greek village lifestyle, all for free. Scan the QR code and enter the information to receive the menu via email!

You can also email me and expect a response as I reply to all emails that I receive! stratisc@evo3oliveoil.com

Also, remember to visit my website at www.evo3oliveoil.com.

And to leave you with one last thought, there is NOTHING as powerful as a changed mind. You can change your hair, your clothing, your address, your spouse, your friends, but if you don't change your mind, the same experience will perpetuate itself over and over again because everything outwardly has changed but nothing inwardly has changed. Once a changed mind has taken hold, a changed life will emerge.

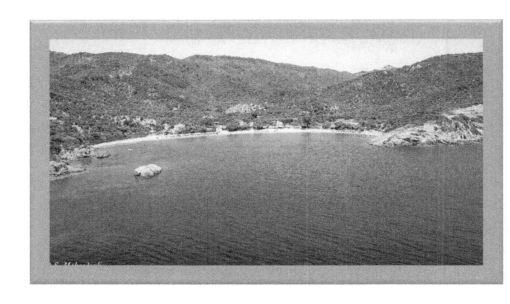

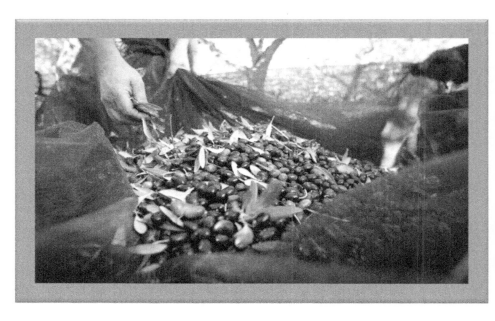

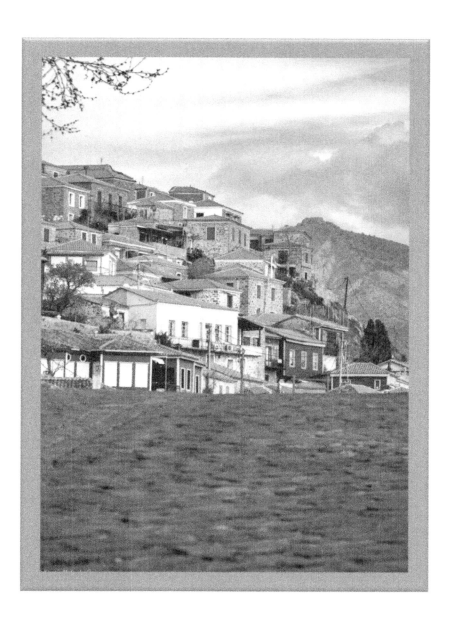

Printed in Great Britain
by Amazon

85936548R00081